Peter Lupus'
Celebrity Body Book:
A Body-Improvement Guide
For Men and Women

By Peter Lupus and Samuel Homola:

Peter Lupus' Guide to Radiant Health and Beauty: Mission Possible for Women

By Samuel Homola:

Bonesetting, Chiropractic, and Cultism

Backache: Home Treatment and Prevention

Muscle Training for Athletes

A Chiropractor's Treasury of Health Secrets

La Salud y Sus Secretos

Secrets of Naturally Youthful Health and Vitality

Doctor Homola's Natural Health Remedies

Remedios Naturales de Salud

Doctor Homola's Life-Extender Health Guide

Doctor Homola's Fat-Disintegrator Diet

Peter Lupus' Celebrity Body Book: A Body-Improvement Guide For Men and Women

by

Peter Lupus and Samuel Homola, D.C.

FOREWORD BY FRANK CAPRIO, M.D.

PARKER PUBLISHING COMPANY, INC.
WEST NYACK, NEW YORK

Library of Congress Cataloging in Publication Data

Lupus, Peter,
    Peter Lupus' celebrity body book.

    Includes index.
    1. Health. 2. Entertainers—Health and
hygiene. I. Homola, Samuel, joint author.
II. Title. III. Title: Celebrity body book.
RA776.5.L88   613   79-27031
ISBN 0-13-661926-6

Dedication

It gives me great pleasure to dedicate this book to the three women who "light up my life" with their love, understanding, and encouragement.

To my mother, Mary Lupus, who helped me get it all started.

To my sister, Rosemary Quillin, who helps keep my head out of the clouds.

To my wife, Sharon Marie, who brought joy and Peter, III into my life.

PETER LUPUS

Credits

Photos by Bill Baldwin, courtesy of "Peter Lupus' Body Shop" television show, Davilup Corporation, Beverly Hills, California.

Foreword by a Doctor of Medicine

This is the second time I have written a foreword for a book by Peter Lupus and Dr. Samuel Homola. When I wrote the foreword for the first book, *Peter Lupus' Guide to Radiant Health and Beauty: Mission Possible for Women,* I complimented the authors for preparing a well-written, medically sound book that was packed with useful information for women. The book was a winner, and it turned out to be one of the most useful and practical health guides ever written exclusively for women.

With this latest book, *Peter Lupus' Celebrity Body Book: A Body-Improvement Guide for Men and Women,* Mr. Lupus and Dr. Homola have surpassed their first book. And in preparing a "body book" that can be used by both men and women, they have greatly broadened their scope of readers.

As the author of 30 self-help books and the director of the Florida Association for Self Improvement, I am always interested in books that laymen can use to improve their mental and physical health. This body-improvement guide by Lupus and Homola is the best I have seen for building and maintaining a strong and healthy body. Their chapters on exercise offer safe and sensible training programs that can be followed by anyone. Other chapters offer health tips on how to care for every portion of the body. The authors tell the reader how to prevent disease, how to relieve the symptoms of common ailments, how to handle physical problems, and how to look better and feel better.

The book is sprinkled throughout with quotations from health-conscious stars and celebrities, many of whom have appeared on Peter Lupus' television show. The celebrity material alone provides exciting reading as well as useful information.

I enthusiastically recommended the first book by Lupus and Homola. I'm even more enthusiastic about this second book by these two authors. I sincerely believe that it will prove to be the best "body book" on the market. If you follow the programs outlined by the authors, you'll certainly improve your health and your physical appearance. So do as I plan to do and add this exciting new book to your health library.

FRANK S. CAPRIO, M.D.
Fort Lauderdale, Florida

What This Book Can Do for You

No one is more concerned about health and physical appearance than a celebrity who is in the public spotlight. In addition to looking good, a celebrity must have good health and considerable endurance to withstand the strain of performing long hours on a hectic schedule. For this reason, most celebrities, especially film actors, are health conscious, and they usually make a special effort to stay strong and healthy. Practically every celebrity we know follows a health program of some kind.

We, the authors, a doctor and an actor, are acquainted with many celebrities. We have had considerable experience in advising celebrities and other people in the formulation of personal health programs. In a special effort to help you develop your own program, we have combined our knowledge and experience with information obtained from interviews with well-known celebrities and health experts who are famous for their health habits. All of this backed up by scientific studies in the field of health forms the basis of the *Peter Lupus Body-Improvement Program* outlined in this book.

YOU CAN LOOK AND FEEL
LIKE A CELEBRITY

You don't have to be a celebrity to look like a celebrity. We all want to feel better, look better, and live longer, and we want to achieve these goals with the easiest, most effective methods available to us. Celebrities who follow a health program have learned from experience how to get the most out of the limited amount of time that a busy schedule allows for a personal health and body-care program. So who would know better than a celebrity how to get the best possible results in the shortest possible time?

Even if you never step on a stage or stand before movie or television cameras, you can benefit from better health and a better body. There's no better way to accomplish this than to follow the same type of program used by celebrities. You don't have to have money or special equipment to follow such programs. All you need is a little knowledge and a little guidance.

HELP FROM FAMOUS CELEBRITIES
IN DEVELOPING YOUR OWN PROGRAM

This book is filled with comments and suggestions obtained from health-conscious celebrities. You'll find them interesting as well as helpful in developing your own body-improvement program. You can learn from the examples of dozens of stars and celebrities who have revealed their health-and-beauty secrets in this book. *Descriptions of the actual programs followed by famous stars provide a wealth of original and useful information for health-conscious readers.*

In outlining the programs covered in the various chapters of this book, we have made a special effort to recommend safe procedures. But if you have a health problem, you should consult a physician. Remember, however, that your health and physical appearance are *your* responsibility. *You* must learn how to take care of yourself if you want to be truly healthy. If you are knowledgeable and well informed about caring for your body, you may know more about some aspects of health than a physician who is concerned only with treating disease. You must depend upon good medical care when you are ill, but maintaining health, preventing disease, and building an attractive body depend primarily upon self help.

SELF HELP IS THE
SECRET OF GOOD HEALTH

With this book, you'll receive the guidance and acquire the knowledge you need to improve the health and appearance of your body with a safe and effective program. And when you don't want to be slowed by aches and pains and common ailments, you can follow our instructions in using self-help procedures to relieve your symptoms and speed your recovery.

Remember that your body is *you.* You can be ugly, weak, and sick, or you can be beautiful, strong, and healthy. It's up to you. With a good body, you'll be happier and more successful—and you'll feel good about yourself. You'll be filled with energy and self-confidence. Best of all, your sex life will be enhanced, and you'll be physically and mentally active long after the average person has fallen by the wayside.

PETER LUPUS
SAMUEL HOMOLA, D.C.

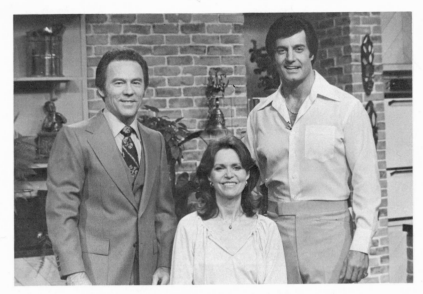

The authors, Dr. Samuel Homola and Peter Lupus,
interview actress and health enthusiast Barbara Feldon,
who is best known for her role as Agent 99 in the "Get
Smart" television series.

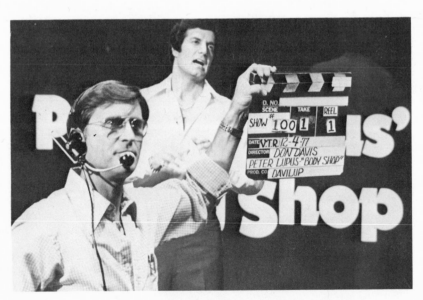

Peter Lupus' Celebrity Body Book is based largely upon
the subject matter of "Peter Lupus' Body Shop" television
series.

Contents

CONTENTS

1

How Celebrities Stay Consistently Slim and Energetic with Body Care

When *John Travolta* signed for the movie "Saturday Night Fever," he began an intensive body-improvement program to prepare himself physically for the performance of rigorous dance scenes. He had to trim excess body fat and condition his muscles—and he had to do so in a hurry. *He lost 25 pounds in two months* following a program that combined diet and exercise with food supplements. He greatly improved his health and his physical appearance, and he increased his energy level as well. He accomplished this by eating such natural foods as broiled or baked lean meat, fish, or chicken, fresh vegetables, and whole wheat bread while taking regular exercise. Between-meal snacks consisted of fresh fruits and juices. Calorie intake was limited to about 2,000 calories a day, and meals were supplemented with a daily multiple vitamin and mineral tablet. In addition to dancing lessons and dance rehearsals, Travolta spent at least half an hour each morning jumping rope, performing calisthenics, or running.

You don't need to exercise as strenuously as John Travolta did unless you want to lose weight in a hurry or prepare for a demanding physical performance. But you should do as he did and combine diet and exercise for the best possible improvement in your physical appearance. And you should eat sensibly in order to protect your health.

Shelly Winters recently lost 30 pounds on the type of diet we recommend. On a balanced diet of fresh fruit, fish, meat, eggs, and milk, supplemented with vitamins and minerals, *she lost a pound a day for a month eating five small meals a day.*

Hard-working stars like John Travolta and Shelly Winters, who must be alert and energetic to keep up their grueling schedules, cannot afford to go on diets that deprive their bodies of essential nutrients. You cannot afford to deprive your body, either, if you want to look good and feel good. You *must* avoid fad diets if you want to protect your health. You should follow the example of celebrities who keep themselves slim and energetic with diet and exercise methods that increase energy as well as improve health and physical appearance.

THE DANGERS OF FAD DIETS

Fad reducing diets can kill you! Yet, most popular reducing diets are fad diets. Promising weight loss overnight, such diets often prove to be too appealing to resist. Many of these diets do result in rapid weight loss, but health often declines as rapidly as body weight diminishes. Starvation or fasting, for example, results in muscle weakness and hair loss from lack of adequate protein. A strict protein or meat-and-water diet drains calcium, potassium, and other essential minerals from your body, resulting in loose teeth or heart trouble. A low-carbohydrate diet that restricts fruits and vegetables deprives the bowels of adequate fiber, resulting in constipation and other problems. A strictly vegetarian diet can lead to the development of anemia. An eat-all-the-fat-you-want diet can clog your arteries and contribute to the development of cancer, and so on.

Specialized diets that restrict the use of any of the basic foods often fail to supply all the nutrients your body needs for good health and a long life. You cannot stay on such diets for very long, and when they are discontinued the lost weight quickly returns. Worst of all, damage to your body may trigger a chain of events that could result in a rapid decline in health. So what should you do to lose weight safely and improve your physical appearance?

THE SECRET: COMBINING DIET AND EXERCISE

In advising actors and celebrities who must look good and feel good to meet the demands of their profession, we have devised a reducing program that assures good health as well as a better-looking body. This program *combines* diet and exercise. If you follow the dietary suggestions offered in this chapter, however, you won't have to exercise strenuously. In fact, you may not have to exercise any more than 15 or 20 minutes every other day to get the benefits you need for a lean, fit body. Best of all, you can eat generously. And the more exercise you take the more you can eat. If you don't exercise, you would have to reduce your food intake so drastically that you may have difficulty getting the nutrients you need for good health.

Your body needs about 1,500 calories a day simply to carry on its basic functions. Generally, you must take in about 15 calories for each pound of body weight each day to maintain your *existing* weight. When you are so inactive that you cannot lose excess fat on a diet that supplies around 2,000 calories a day, you cannot possibly build and maintain a truly beautiful and healthy body.

The fewer calories you take in the more weight you lose, especially when you exercise. Most nutritionists feel, however, that a diet that supplies fewer than 1,200 calories a day is deficient in essential nutrients. There's no doubt that it is difficult for the average woman to get adequate iron on a diet that supplies no more than 2,000 calories. There is some evidence to indicate that it may take at least 3,000 natural-food calories a day to assure an adequate intake of *all* the essential nutrients. So rather than attempt to lose weight rapidly on a low-calorie diet, it would be best to lose gradually on a generous diet that is combined with an exercise program, especially if you want an attractive body molded by well-developed muscles. Besides, if you eat strictly natural foods, you'll find that you can eat all you want and still lose excess body fat.

TV actress *Shannon Wilcox* burns calories and develops her muscles with resistive exercise provided by a Nautilus machine. This allows her to take in considerably more than 2,000 calories a day, supplying all the nutrients she needs for good health and a beautiful body.

Movie actor James Hampton and actress Shannon Wilcox both recommend a combination of diet and exercise to control body weight.

BALANCING MUSCLE AND FAT

Unless you have a medical problem and your doctor puts you on a special fasting diet, don't try to lose more than a couple of pounds a week by cutting calories. Weight lost slowly on a good diet is less likely to come back than weight lost rapidly on a fasting diet. Also, the type of diet you need to supply adequate nutrients for your body won't allow overly rapid weight loss. A pound a week adds up to 52 pounds a year—and that's fast enough for most people.

Many overweight people can lose three or four pounds of fat a week simply by switching to a diet of natural foods, even if they eat generously and don't exercise. Weight loss can be speeded by endurance-type exercises, but muscle-building exercises may temporarily slow weight loss. The reason for this is that as you develop the muscles of your body, muscle weight will replace fat loss. With continued loss of fat, however, your weight will soon begin to drop. When fat is reduced to a normal level, your muscular development will reward you with a shapely body.

How do you know when you have a normal amount of fat? If you can pinch up more than one inch of fat anywhere on your body, you have too much fat. If you *look* fat when you stand nude in front of a mirror, you *are* fat, regardless of what the scales say. Be careful, however, not to mistake flabby muscles for fat. If you look thin but flabby, you may need to do muscle-building exercises. Inactive persons who try to diet away flab without exercising may eventually reduce down to a skinny but still-flabby body. You must have "meat" on your bones to have an attractive body. And this means having more muscle than fat—whether you are a man or a woman.

As long as you have fat to lose, continue with the type of exercise recommended in Chapter 2. If you want to gain weight or build your muscles, do the exercises described in Chapter 3. In either case, stick to the basic dietary rules outlined in this chapter.

THE NATURAL FOODS PROGRAM
FOR WEIGHT CONTROL

When you combine diet with a moderate amount of exercise and follow the instructions outlined in this chapter, you don't have to worry about counting calories. *All you have to do is restrict your diet to the use of certain types of foods.* This way, with diet and exercise, you can use a moderate approach in the use of both measures. You'll be able to eat enough to enjoy eating, and you won't have to torture yourself with an excessive amount of exercise. (If you want to count calories for rapid weight loss without exercising, read *Doctor Homola's Fat-Disintegrator Diet,* Parker Publishing Company.)

Even if you lose weight following the basic rules outlined in this chapter, remember that it's still important to exercise regularly if you want a really good-looking body. Losing fat without toning or developing your muscles may not greatly improve the appearance of your body.

When movie actor and singer *Gordon MacRae* appeared on "Body Shop," the diet and exercise hints he picked up from home economist *Sybil Henderson* and exercise expert *Peter Lupus* contributed to his weight loss, resulting in Gordon's new, trim waistline.

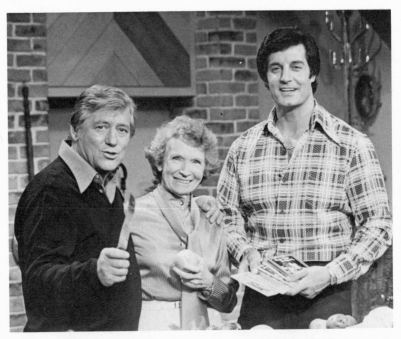

Singer Gordon MacRae and home economist Sybil Henderson believe that low-calorie cooking should supply all of the essential nutrients.

Basic Rules for Healthful Loss of Body Fat

Here are the basic rules you'll be following on your celebrity reducing diet. Once you understand how to carry out the recommendations underlying these rules, you may simply pin a copy of the rules on your kitchen wall or carry them in your pocket for daily use. You must study the remainder of this chapter, however, in order to get the guidance you need to follow these rules effectively.

1. Do not use sugar or eat foods containing sugar or white flour.
2. Do not eat processed foods or snacks.
3. Eat lean meats, skinned poultry, fish, eggs, fresh fruits and vegetables, raw salads, cottage cheese and yogurt made from skimmed milk, and whole-grain breads and cereals.
4. Do not use fats or oils in cooking.
5. Increase the amount of fiber in your diet by adding unprocessed miller's bran to cereals and other foods.
6. Use skimmed milk, unsweetened juices, and water as beverages. Drink *water* when you are thirsty.
7. Use one tablespoon of cold-pressed vegetable oil on a green salad each day.
8. Eat slowly at mealtime. Stop eating when you are comfortably full.
9. Satisfy your craving for sweets by eating fresh and dried fruits for dessert following meals.
10. If you feel hungry, shaky, or weak between meals, snack on baked chicken or a little plain yogurt or uncreamed cottage cheese with a piece of fresh fruit.

Will these simple rules work for you? Yes!

Harriet B. wrote to tell us that she lost 15 pounds in one month following these basic rules. "That's the best diet I've ever been on," she raved. "As long as I follow your basic rules, I eat as much as I want when I get hungry and the fat just keeps disappearing."

Johnny T. lost only a pound or two a week following the basic rules. "But I'm not complaining," he told us. "I started the diet six months ago and I'm still losing weight. So far, I've lost 25 pounds. And I look better and feel better than ever before in my life!"

Begin by Eliminating
Refined Sugar from Your Diet

The average American consumes about 125 pounds of sugar a

year! Nothing is more fattening than sugar. Most people who are overweight could lose weight simply by eliminating sugar from their diet. This isn't always easy to do, however, unless you prepare all of your foods from scratch. Practically all processed foods contain sugar. The catsup you use on your hamburger, for example, contains sugar. Even the canned vegetables you buy often contain sugar. So it's not enough to remove the sugar bowl from your dinner table. You must eat at home and prepare your own foods so that you can rest assured that they are fresh and nutritious as well as free from sugar.

If you must use a sweetener occasionally, try using honey, brown sugar, or molasses. Although these sweeteners are high in calories and must be used sparingly, they contain traces of chromium and other nutrients that help protect your body against the adverse effects of sugar. Since honey is actually sweeter than sugar, you'll use less honey than sugar as a sweetener. You'll also find that honey satisfies your craving for sweets much better than sugar.

Molasses is rich in iron, calcium, and the B vitamins you need to metabolize sugar. White sugar contains nothing but calories. In fact, when you eat white sugar, it actually *steals* nutrients from your body. Sugar also stimulates the production of insulin by your pancreas. When your pancreas has been overworked and sensitized by excessive use of sugar, the use of only a small amount of sugar (or any sweetener) can result in a pancreatic overreaction that can cause a *fall* in blood sugar a few hours later. This forces your body to store blood sugar as glycogen (which may then be converted to fat), leaving you tired, hungry, and shaky with a craving for sweets. Furthermore, the depletion of B vitamins and other nutrients used in the metabolism of sugar lowers the metabolic efficiency of your body. This is one reason why the calories supplied by sugar are more fattening than the calories supplied by natural foods.

Obviously, if you are overweight, you cannot afford to use even a small amount of sugar. Even if you aren't overweight, you should use sugar sparingly, if at all, in order to protect your health. It is now well known that excessive use of sugar contributes to the development of a great variety of diseases. In addition to increasing blood levels of cholesterol and triglycerides, for example, sugar contributes to the development of colon cancer by altering the bacterial content of the bowel.

Your body does not need the empty calories supplied by sugar. *Forcing* your body to metabolize sugar can lead to the development of diabetes and other body-killing diseases. Most celebrities who follow a health program avoid the use of sugar; it is certainly not used in the *Peter Lupus Body-Improvement Program*. Ask any health-conscious celebrity about using sugar and chances are you'll be advised to eliminate it completely. *Muhammad Ali,* for example, learned from comedian *Dick Gregory* that sugar can harm the body. "Dick Gregory has gotten me off all white sugar and sodas," says Muhammad. "When I'm in training now, I need a room just for my vitamins."

Gloria Swanson is Hollywood's most vocal opponent of sugar. "That stuff is poison," she maintains. "I won't have it in my house, let alone in my body." Her influence in helping *William Dufty* kick the sugar habit led to a miraculous transformation in his health and physical appearance and to publication of his best-selling book *Sugar Blues.*

White Flour Should Be Eliminated, Too!

Like sugar, white flour is a refined carbohydrate. Excessive use of white-flour products can trigger a blood-sugar reaction that may make it impossible for you to lose weight. Even a small amount of white flour can make a low-calorie diet ineffective. For this reason, white flour and its products, like sugar, should be totally eliminated from your diet if you are overweight. Many processed foods contain white flour as well as sugar. So be sure to stick to the use of fresh, natural foods when preparing your meals.

The carbohydrate found in whole-grain products and fresh fruits and vegetables is a *complex* carbohydrate that is not nearly as fattening as the simple carbohydrate found in refined foods. As you'll learn later in this chapter, you can actually use fiber-rich natural carbohydrate to help you *lose* weight!

Note: When you use flour at home, use whole-grain wheat, rye, or soya flour—or use corn meal.

How to Recognize Processed Foods

Processed foods are usually rich in simple carbohydrate and deficient in fiber and essential nutrients. They may also contain artificial additives as well as sugar. Since processed foods can be manufactured in great quantities and won't easily spoil, they are more profitable to sell. This is why television advertising is usually devoted to the sale of processed foods rather than to the sale of fresh, natural foods.

Any packaged food that doesn't resemble its natural food source or is heavily sugared or salted should be avoided whenever possible. The processed snacks in boxes that line the shelves of supermarkets should not even be sampled. It's difficult to resist these snacks when you are hungry. Try to do your grocery shopping *after* you have eaten so that you won't be tempted by junk foods.

Read the Labels on Packaged Foods

When you do shop for packaged foods, be sure to read the labels before you buy. If the food does not contain all-natural ingredients, do not buy it. Remember, however, that some food manufacturers classify sugar as a natural ingredient. If you are overweight, you should not eat any food that has been sweetened with sugar.

Frozen and canned foods may be all right if their labels do not indicate that they contain added sugar, preservatives, or fat. Sugar is sometimes referred to as sucrose, glucose, or dextrose, while fat might be represented with such terms as hydrogenated vegetable oil, monoglycerides, and diglycerides. So unless you are an experienced label reader, you should try to select fresh, natural foods when you go grocery shopping. For example, choose real potatoes instead of powdered potatoes, brown rice instead of white rice, whole-grain bread instead of white bread, fresh vegetables instead of canned or frozen vegetables, fresh meats instead of lunch meats, orange juice instead of "orange drink," and so on. Any modern supermarket can supply you with all the natural foods you need for a balanced diet.

Superhealthy *Jack La Lanne* (best known for his television exercise program) recommends natural foods. He offers us this advice about diet: "Eating foods as close to their natural state as possible sums up my philosophy about nutrition. If man makes it, don't eat it. Be sure that bread is 100 percent whole wheat. Include lots of fresh fruits and vegetables, especially leafy vegetables, in your diet. Chicken is high on my list, too. Avoid white flour and sugars completely."

Today, at the age of 65, Jack La Lanne pays as much attention to his diet as he does to his exercise program—and he is in great shape. He confides that he plans to celebrate his next birthday by walking one mile up Hollywood Boulevard while supporting a 350-pound barbell across his shoulders!

Arnold Schwarzenegger, a former "Mr. Universe" who recently received the Golden Globe Award as the best new actor and who is presently starring in the movie "The Villain," echos La Lanne's philosophy when it comes to eating nutritious natural foods. "A good diet means nothing if the foods are not *fresh,*" Arnold insists. His performance in "The Villain" has proved that Arnold has talent as well as muscles.

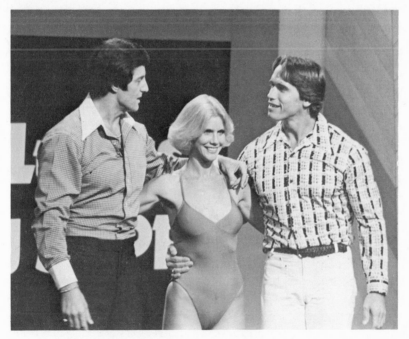

*"Mr. Universe" Arnold Schwarzenegger (right), actress
Shannon Wilcox, and "Body Shop" host Peter Lupus feed
their bodies with fresh, natural foods.*

Complex Carbohydrates
Are Essential for Good Health

While you should avoid refined carbohydrates as much as possible, don't succumb to the promises of zero-carbohydrate diets.

You *must* have 100 grams or more of natural (complex) carbohydrate in your diet each day for the best of health. Your body needs the fiber and the micronutrients supplied by natural carbohydrate foods. It's the refined carbohydrate that you don't need. It's not likely that you can get fat eating such natural carbohydrates as fresh fruits, vegetables, potatoes, and whole-grain products. As we noted earlier, there is now some evidence to indicate that eating natural carbohydrate foods that are rich in fiber may even help you *reduce* your bodyweight. The high-fiber content of coarse whole-grain products actually interferes with absorption of calories. And the coarser the product the fewer the calories absorbed. You may even be able to *speed* weight loss by including a variety of coarse whole-grain products in your diet.

Remember that raw fruits and vegetables are complex carbohydrates, and they are rich in cellulose (a form of fiber). Be sure to include them in your food selections each day—whether you are overweight or not.

HOW TO SELECT BASIC FOODS
FOR BODY IMPROVEMENT

You can simplify selection of basic foods for your body-improvement program by making a list of the various food groups and then selecting at least one food from each group every day. In the meat group, for example, you can select from lean meats, skinned poultry, fish, or eggs. If you eat meat, it's very important to cut away all visible fat. It is presently the consensus among medical men that animal fat contributes to the development of cardiovascular disease. There is also some evidence to indicate that animal fat might be a cause of cancer! So whether you are overweight or not, you should cut down on consumption of beef and pork and eat more fish and poultry.

You may eat generous amounts of all types of vegetables as long as they are raw or cooked without grease or oil. Fruits, of course, should always be eaten raw.

Raw salads made from fresh fruits and vegetables and served with uncreamed cottage cheese or yogurt made from skimmed milk will provide a nutritious meal for overweight dieters.

Skimmed milk and its products (such as cheese) are good sources of protein as well as calcium. If you are intolerant to lactose (milk sugar), use *fermented* milk products.

Raw fruits and vegetables supply fiber as well as Vitamin C. You should, however, make sure that your diet includes whole-grain breads and cereals for their Vitamin E, magnesium, zinc, selenium, and B vitamins as well as for their fiber. Bran flakes, granola, oats, shredded wheat, and wheat germ are good examples of natural (whole-grain) cereals. You should, of course, avoid refined or sugar-sweetened cereals. When you need a sweetener for your cereal, use honey or raisins.

Note: When you buy cereals that require cooking, such as grits, oatmeal, or rice, don't buy the instant or quick-cooking variety. Such cereals contain less fiber and fewer nutrients than their longer-cooking counterparts.

The Seven Basic Food Groups

Here are the basic food groups you should choose from:

1. Green and yellow vegetables
2. Citrus fruit, tomatoes, and raw cabbage
3. Potatoes and other vegetables and fruits
4. Skimmed milk and skimmed milk products
5. Lean meat, skinned poultry, fish, eggs, and dried peas and beans
6. Whole-grain breads, cereals, and flours
7. Vegetable oil and butter

Make sure that you eat something from each of these groups every day. Select fresh, natural foods whenever possible. Turn to Chapter 10 for instructions in how to prepare these foods for maximum nutrients and minimum calories.

Dinah Shore follows sensible guidelines in selecting foods for a reducing diet. "My idea of a health food is a *fresh* food," she explained in discussing her preference for natural foods. "Vegetables are best when they're dark green and leafy; they have the most vitamins. I don't believe in crash dieting—you lose too many precious nutrients. When I'm overweight, I just eat *less* of everything. That way, I get proper nutrition and I don't feel tired."

Marie Osmond of the "Donny and Marie" television show was 46 pounds overweight when she was 10 years old. Today, at the age of 19, she is beautiful and slim. How does she do it? We know that she gets plenty of exercise rehearsing and performing dance routines. She also plays golf and tennis. Here is how she describes her diet: "I eat nutritious food and never skip a meal. I like lean meat or fish, salads, and fruit juices at lunchtime. At dinner, I'll eat lean meat, vegetables, and bread. I drink skim milk with my dinner."

Marie gives her mother credit for her successful fight against obesity. "I've given you the basics," she says her mother always told her. "If you eat the way you've been raised to eat, without all of the junk foods you used to eat outside the home, you'll never have to worry about your weight again."

This chapter also gives you the basics. If you follow its guidelines, you'll never have to worry, either, about your weight!

HOW TO ADD BODY-CLEANING FIBER
TO YOUR FOODS

In addition to helping you reduce or control your body weight, plenty of fiber in your diet will also help prevent constipation, hemorrhoids, diverticular disease, colon cancer, gallstones, and atherosclerosis. Colon cancer is presently the second most common cause of death from cancer, following close behind lung cancer. Medical scientists now believe that lack of adequate fiber in the diet is a major cause of colon cancer. (For an explanation, see Chapter 8.) So even if you aren't overweight, you should make sure that your diet includes plenty of fiber-rich natural foods.

You can add additional fiber to your diet by sprinkling unprocessed miller's bran over the foods you eat. Bran can be added to cereals, for example, or it can be mixed into meat loaf, homemade bread, casseroles, and other appropriate dishes. Since bran is indigestible, it simply passes through your digestive tract, absorbing water to produce a zero-calorie bulk that sweeps your bowel clean.

How to Take Bran

If you're overweight, you might want to take two teaspoons of bran with a glass of water before each meal in order to curb your

TV comedian and actor *Dave Madden* of "Laugh-In" fame, like many Hollywood stars, must work on a rigid schedule. Dave says that he works best on a fiber-rich diet that keeps his intestinal tract healthy, regular, and dependable.

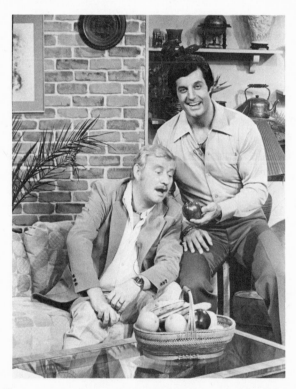

That apple really tempts comedian Dave Madden, since he regularly eats fresh fruits and vegetables to enrich his diet with fiber.

appetite. The absorbent bran will swell in your stomach to produce a sensation of fullness. It's generally best, however, to add bran to foods during regular meals.

Don't worry about bran being too coarse for your bowels. Bran is actually so soft that some doctors call it "softage" rather than roughage.

Too much bran in your diet might be harmful; so don't overdo it.

Since bran can interfere with absorption of calories, it might also interfere with absorption of nutrients. Adding an excessive amount of miller's bran to your diet might lead to a deficiency in iron, zinc, calcium, and other minerals. You should never go on a reducing diet that consists only of bran and water. Just add a couple of teaspoons of bran to each meal and then eat less. As you become accustomed to using bran, you may increase the amount you use—provided you add it to foods or use it as a supplement to a balanced diet. You can't get too much bran from natural foods, so continue to eat as many fiber-rich foods as you can.

In determining how much miller's bran you should take, be guided by the nature of your bowel movements. When you experience regular movements with well-formed, moist stools, you are taking adequate bran.

Unprocessed miller's bran is very inexpensive and can be purchased in any health food store. It has a pleasant whole-grain taste and can be used to enhance the flavor of a variety of dishes. You'll learn in other chapters of this book how bran and other forms of fiber actually help prevent the development of many common diseases. Be sure to read every chapter of this book if you really want to do all you can for your body.

BE CAREFUL ABOUT WHAT YOU DRINK!

What you drink can be just as important as what you eat when it comes to taking care of your body. You already know that excessive use of sugar can be harmful to your body. Do you know that companies manufacturing soft-drink beverages in America use more sugar than any other single industry? According to recent marketing research figures, *Americans consume more soft drinks than any other beverage*—34.2 gallons per person each year! That adds up to a large amount of sugar.

Coffee is second on the list of favorite American beverages, followed by milk, beer, and tea.

Simply avoiding soft drinks would greatly reduce sugar consumption. Even if you drink artificially sweetened beverages, the artificial colors, flavors, preservatives, and other additives, including the sweetener, may be harmful to your body. So stay away from soft drinks, even if they aren't sweetened with sugar.

Many people use a couple teaspoons of sugar in a cup of coffee—and they may drink several cups of coffee a day. Sugar intake could be greatly reduced among coffee drinkers simply by getting rid of the sugar bowl. Like soft drinks, however, coffee is bad for you with or without sugar. The caffeine in coffee, for example, is a common cause of headache, nervousness, and irritability. Worst of all for the overweight person, caffeine can trigger hypoglycemia (low blood sugar) by stimulating the adrenal glands, resulting in forced storage of blood sugar as fat. Overweight persons who have trouble losing weight on a low-calorie diet should avoid coffee as well as sugar and white flour. Tea also contains caffeine. So do colas.

If you want to be good to your body, drink *water* when you are thirsty. You need plenty of water to form bulk from the fiber in the foods you eat. Remember rule No. 6: Use water, skimmed milk, or unsweetened juices as beverages with your meals. Avoid coffee, tea, and soft drinks.

HOW TO USE VEGETABLE OIL
FOR BETTER HEALTH

In rule No. 7, you were advised to use one tablespoon of cold-pressed vegetable oil on a green salad each day. You must have a certain amount of soft vegetable oil in your diet to balance the hard animal fat in your foods. Since you'll be cutting down on your consumption of animal fat on the *Peter Lupus Body-Improvement Program,* you won't need to add more than one or two tablespoons of vegetable oil to your diet each day.

There is now some evidence to indicate that too much vegetable oil, like too much animal fat, can contribute to the development of cancer. Oxidation of fatty acids in the body forms dangerous peroxides and depletes Vitamin E reserves. Vegetable oils normally contain Vitamin E, but when they are processed they do not retain adequate amounts of this important vitamin. You must have Vitamin E to prevent oxidation of fatty acids. So the more vegetable oil you use the more Vitamin E you need.

Movie actor *James Hampton,* who performed recently in "China Syndrome," includes cooking among his hobbies, but he is careful about the amount and type of fat he consumes.

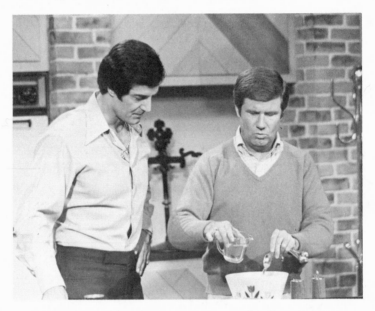

Movie actor James Hampton, star of "Cat From Outer Space," uses cold-pressed vegetable oil in his cooking in order to balance his diet with essential fatty acids.

If you cut down on your intake of animal fat and limit your use of vegetable oil to a couple of tablespoons daily, and then supplement your diet with a few hundred units of Vitamin E, you'll lose weight as well as combat cancer.

Note: Do not depend upon heated vegetable oils for your essential fatty acids. When vegetable oil is heated to temperatures above 215 degrees centigrade (419 degrees Fahrenheit) for 15 minutes or longer, the fatty acids are broken down into a toxic substance. It's okay to use a little cold-pressed vegetable oil on a green salad, but you should not use fats or oils in cooking.

Remember that margarine, though made from vegetable oil, has been converted to a saturated fat that is similar to animal fat. So don't try to substitute margarine for vegetable oil to get your essential fatty acids.

PUT YOUR APPETITIE MECHANISM TO WORK

When you eat properly, your appetitie mechanism will usually let you know when you have had enough to eat. Properly prepared natural foods, for example, will provide low-calorie bulk that will readily satisfy your appetite. Best of all, when you eliminate sugar and white-flour products from your diet and stick to natural foods, you won't experience the blood sugar fluctuations that result in excessive craving or a stubborn appetite.

It's really very difficult to overeat or gain weight when you limit your diet to lean meats, fresh fruits and vegetables, and other basic foods. Even potatoes are not fattening when they are properly prepared. Natural carbohydrates won't artificially stimulate your appetite. And once you eliminate refined carbohydrates from your diet, you'll be able to eat more and still lose weight.

"For years I ate junk food," tennis star *Billie Jean King* admitted recently, "but now I'm on a new program of fish, fresh fruit, and vegetables and I'm finally keeping my weight down."

You can, too, if you eat properly.

Don't Rush Your Stomach

Your weight will automatically adjust itself at a level that is best for you when you eat properly and exercise regularly. It's important, however, to eat slowly in order to give your body time to absorb nutrients and raise your blood sugar enough to satisfy the appetite centers in your brain. Always stop eating when you are comfortably full. Try to get up from the table feeling that you could eat a little more.

Remember that no matter how full your stomach is, your hunger won't be fully satisfied until nutrients circulating in your blood reach the appetite centers in your brain. This means that if you eat slowly and get up from the table a little hungry, you won't be hungry an hour later. So don't hurriedly stuff your stomach in an attempt to quickly satisfy your hunger.

GIVE YOUR SWEET TOOTH A BREAK

Although you should try to quit eating candy and other commercial sweets, few of us want to deprive ourselves of the pleasure of eating something sweet occasionally. Actually, you can *benefit* from eating such nutritious natural sweets as fresh and dried fruits. With a little imagination, you can prepare homemade sweets that are healthful as well as tasty. Whenever possible, however, try to satisfy your sweet tooth with fresh or dried fruits. A piece of fruit with cheese makes a satisfying dessert.

Fresh fruit can be eaten any time, even between meals. But when you eat dried fruits or homemade sweets, reserve them for desserts following meals. This way you won't spoil your appetite for basic foods and your blood sugar won't be disturbed. Once your appetite has been satisfied with a balanced meal, your craving for sweets will diminish or disappear.

Make sure that the sweets you eat are natural and nourishing. There are a variety of healthful, *natural* sweets that you can serve to friends as well as to your family. Take a look in your local health food store.

EAT FIVE TIMES A DAY!

Many people on a reducing diet make the mistake of eating only one meal a day, hoping to reduce their body weight by cutting down their calorie intake. What usually happens, though, is that hunger created by an empty stomach and a fall in blood sugar results in an uncontrollable urge to overeat. Sudden loading of the stomach and the resulting sudden rise in blood sugar then stimulates the storage of body fat. It would be much better to eat four or five small meals than one large meal. This way, the level of sugar and nutrients in your blood will be consistent enough to appease the appetite mechanism in your brain and it won't take much food to satisfy your hunger.

Chances are you'll take in *fewer* calories a day by eating frequent small meals than by eating one large meal. It's essential, of course, that you eat fresh, *natural* foods rather than processed foods in order to avoid artificially stimulating your appetite and triggering a pancreatic reaction.

Persons who suffer from functional hypoglycemia, or recurring low blood sugar, may find it necessary to snack between meals to keep their blood sugar up enough to prevent a craving for sweets and starches. Between-meal snacks should consist of such foods as plain yogurt or uncreamed cottage cheese with fresh fruit. Baked chicken or some other low-fat, high-protein food will maintain a normal blood sugar level. You'll learn more about hypoglycemia in Chapter 9.

MEAL SUBSTITUTES
IN A REDUCING DIET

When it's not convenient to prepare a meal made from the foods you must have to reduce your weight or avoid a weight gain, or when you simply want to eat less without hurting your body, you may occasionally substitute a high-protein milkshake for one or two meals a day. When you do use such a drink you should supplement the drink with multiple vitamins and minerals. This way, you can "fast" without depriving your body of essential nutrients and without forcing your body to burn precious muscle protein for energy. It's very important, however, to eat at least one balanced meal each day in order to get nutrients not supplied by supplements.

It's never a good idea to go on a total fast or to substitute a protein drink for all three meals. Limiting your diet to a protein drink may force your body to excrete calcium, potassium, and other nutrients that are essential for good health and a strong heart. When you cannot eat three meals a day, try to eat *at least* one meal and then fill in temporarily with a good high-protein milkshake that is supplemented with vitamins and minerals.

You'll learn more about how to prepare healthful drinks when you read Chapter 11. And you'll find recipes used by some of your favorite celebrities. In the meantime, you can quickly make a healthful protein drink by mixing a couple tablespoons of protein *powder* with skimmed milk in a blender, adding ice and your favorite fruit or frozen concentrate.

HOW TO USE VITAMIN AND
MINERAL SUPPLEMENTS

There are about 50 nutrients known to be essential for good health, but recommended daily allowances have been established for only about 17 of these. There are undoubtedly many undiscovered

Men and women alike can benefit from the same general health measures, including health drinks. When we interviewed manly screen star *Vic Morrow* along with beautiful model *Maurine Dawson,* we found that both had similar health habits. So whether you are a rugged outdoorsman or a fashion model, you can benefit from the general guidelines of this book.

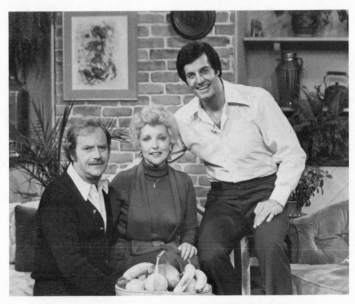

Rugged movie and TV actor Vic Morrow and beauty expert Maurine Dawson share common interests when it comes to use of diet and exercise for better health and an improved physical appearance.

nutrients in natural foods, all of which are probably also essential for good health. So while you should supplement your diet with vitamins and minerals when you are on a low-calorie diet, you must never totally substitute supplements for basic foods.

Except in cases of a deficiency or when you need additional amounts of specific nutrients during periods of stress or illness, you should not arbitrarily dose yourself with large amounts of a single vitamin or mineral. Too much Vitamin A, for example, can be toxic and can result in a need for larger amounts of Vitamin E. Taking large doses of one B vitamin can create a deficiency in other B vitamins. If you suffer from gouty arthritis or kidney stones, large amounts of Vitamin C might aggravate your problem by forming oxalic acid in your body. An overdose of Vitamin D can result in retention of too much calcium in your body. Taking iron with Vitamin E might interfere with absorption of Vitamin E. Too much zinc might raise blood cholesterol by upsetting the ratio of zinc to copper in your body. Iron can be toxic when taken in large doses by persons not suffering from anemia, and so on.

Unless you have a specific problem, just take a good multiple vitamin and mineral supplement when you are on a low-calorie reducing diet.

When you have a deficiency or an increased need for a vitamin or mineral, you can take larger doses in combination with supporting nutrients. Vitamin C, for example, can be taken with bioflavonoids or with orange juice, Vitamin A with Vitamin E, and calcium with Vitamin D. Vitamin B can be taken in a B complex formula, Vitamin E in the form of mixed tocopherols, and so on. When illness strikes, vitamins can be taken in mega doses, that is, in doses larger than those required to correct a simple deficiency. In order to take mega doses of vitamins and minerals safely and effectively, however, you must know what you are doing—or you must have professional guidance.

You'll learn more about how to take vitamins in other chapters of this book. And we'll tell you how our Hollywood friends use supplements along with foods to maintain good health and a high level of energy. In the meantime, just remember to use supplements *after* you have made a special effort to eat properly.

SUMMARY

1. The best way to reduce your body weight and improve your physical appearance is to combine diet and exercise.

2. A healthful reducing diet should be made up of basic natural foods that supply all the essential nutrients you need to feel good and look good.

3. Everyone, overweight or not, should try to eliminate sugar, white-flour products, and other refined carbohydrates from their diet.

4. If you eat properly and exercise regularly, your appetite mechanism will automatically adjust your body weight at a level that is best for you.

5. You may be able to lose weight more rapidly by eating five small meals a day rather than three regular meals or one large meal.

6. You should always take nutritional supplements when you are on a reducing diet.

7. Adding unprocessed miller's bran to your diet will provide zero-calorie bulk as well as aid in maintaining a healthy intestinal tract.

8. Fats and oils should be balanced and reduced to a minimum in order to eliminate excess calories as well as to prevent cancer.

9. Sweets should be limited to fresh and dried fruits with occasional all-natural homemade desserts.

10. When you use protein-powder drinks as a meal substitute, you should eat at least one balanced meal a day and then supplement your diet with vitamins and minerals.

2

Celebrity Exercise Programs For Lasting Fitness

In Chapter 1, you learned that the secret of maintaining a lean, *healthy* body is combining a sensible diet with regular exercise. But don't worry. You don't have to knock yourself out with a marathon exercise program. All it takes is a little recreational exercise three or four times a week.

Whether you are overweight or not, you should exercise regularly. According to a joint 10-year study just released by researchers at Stanford University and the Harvard School of Public Health, Harvard graduates between the ages of 35 and 74 who burned less than 2,000 calories a week with regular exercise had a 64 percent higher risk of heart attack than those who burned *more* than 2,000 calories a week with regular exercise.

It's not difficult to burn 2,000 or more calories a week by exercising. Playing handball or tennis half an hour a day or for a little over one hour every other day, for example, burns about 2,000 calories.

Tennis is a popular form of exercise in Hollywood. The services of Hollywood tennis instructor *Patty Heard,* for example, are in such great demand among film stars that she is referred to as the "tennis pro of the stars."

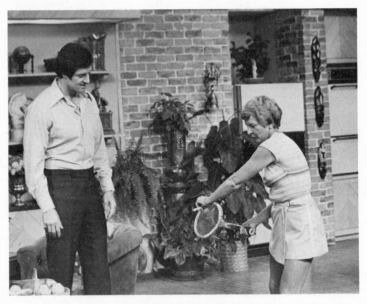

Tennis expert Patty Heard teaches Hollywood stars how to stay fit and develop cardiovascular endurance by playing tennis.

YOU DON'T HAVE TO EXERCISE EVERY DAY!

On a weight-reducing program, it really does not matter how you burn calories. You don't even have to do all of your exercises at one time. You can exercise a few minutes at a time several times a day if you like. You can burn 300 or more calories a day simply by being moderately active. Working in the yard, washing the car, making home repairs, and performing other simple jobs, for example, may be all you'll have to do—provided, of course, that you cut down on your eating. If you want to strengthen your heart, however, you must exercise vigorously enough to get your pulse rate up to about 120 beats per minute (a moderate elevation) and keep it there for a few minutes at least twice a week—preferably every other day.

So while you can burn calories by doing a few simple exercises for only a few minutes several times a day, you should try to participate in some form of endurance-type recreational exercise, such as swimming, bicycling, rope jumping, handball, or tennis, two or three times a week if you want to keep your heart strong.

You must, of course, condition yourself gradually in any endurance-type athletic activity. The secret is to participate regularly, never pushing yourself to the point of distress or discomfort. As time goes by, you'll automatically exercise more as you become better conditioned. Once you are able to perform the exercise continuously without discomfort, you can maintain your pulse rate at 120 beats per minute for several minutes without any trouble whatsoever.

Note: When you first begin exercising, it won't take much more than a brisk walk to get your heart rate up to 120 beats per minute. As you become better conditioned, it'll take more effort to get your heart rate up, but there'll be less discomfort.

Persons seeking a high level of cardiovascular fitness should gradually work up to an exercise program that requires several minutes of warm up preceding 20 to 30 minutes of continuous endurance-type exercise that keeps the heart beating about 75 percent of its maximum capacity, followed by several minutes of gradually decreasing effort. Such exercise should be performed at least every other day for best results.

Maximum heart rates vary for individuals, depending upon age and physical condition. The younger the person, the higher the training heart rate can be—up to about 170 beats per minute. For most of us, a training heart rate of about 120 is a safe, moderate range.

Recommended reading: *Rating the Exercises,* by the Editors of *Consumer Guide,* William Morrow Company.

Keep Your Exercise Comfortable

If you follow the general dietary rules outlined in Chapter 1, and then make an effort to stay moderately active with at least an every-other-day exercise program, you won't have any trouble controlling your body weight. Remember that you can benefit just as much—or more—from frequent, abbreviated exercise programs as from occasional long workouts if all you want to do is reduce your body weight. You don't have to exercise longer than 10 or 15 minutes at a time, and you don't have to go nonstop for hundreds of repetitions. If you want to trim down your waist or tone up your abdominal muscles with sit-ups, for example, you can benefit more by doing 10 or 12 repetitions—or as many as you can comfortably do—three or four times a day rather than by trying to do them all at one time.

Actress and dancer *Elaine Joyce* gets plenty of exercise rehearsing and dancing on Broadway stages, but she still exercises at home as well— and she does so throughout the day at her convenience, in short mini-workouts.

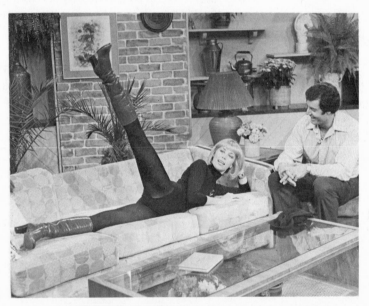

Broadway actress and dancer Elaine Joyce demonstrates a slimming exercise that any housewife can do frequently and comfortably at home.

The point is that you must not torture yourself with exercise so that you dread doing it. Unless you're training for an athletic event, you don't need the strength and endurance of an athlete. You don't have to jog 10 miles or develop a washboard abdomen unless that's what you want or need. With only a small amount of effort, you can keep your waist trim and maintain the ability to jog a mile or two. You can burn an adequate number of calories without even sweating if you exercise frequently enough. But remember that if you want to strengthen your heart muscle and open your blood vessels, you'll have to exercise strenuously enough to *force* your heart to beat fairly rapidly for several minutes at a time.

Whatever type of exercise you do, it should be something that you can do conveniently and comfortably.

Film star Hugh O'Brian, famed as TV's "Wyatt Earp," works his exercise into his daily routine to avoid training boredom. In Hugh's living room, he found his sofa can be used for beneficial push-ups. Such regular exercises have kept him in top physical condition.

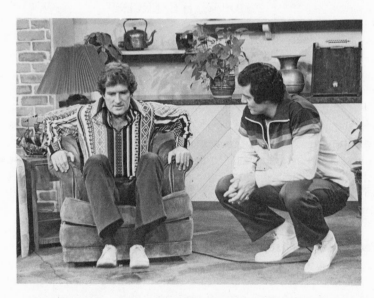

*Hugh O'Brian, the movie Wyatt Earp, does sofa push-ups
at home to keep his arms and shoulders strong.*

Marilyn R. reduced her body weight, improved her physical appearance, and increased her energy simply by exercising a few minutes at a time several times a day in her home. "I work squats, sit-ups, and other basic exercises into my daily routine," Marilyn explained. "I exercise only a few minutes at a time, but the results have been fantastic! Now, instead of driving to the grocery store, I walk. My body has firmed up and my energy and endurance have doubled. Thanks for such a simple alternative to a long, boring workout."

Jack D. prefers jogging, but he avoids overexertion by alternating walking with jogging. "I walk awhile and jog awhile every evening before supper," Jack reported. "I never really exert myself. But I can now jog a mile non-stop without any difficulty—and my pulse rate rarely goes above 120. I feel like a new man! My legs no longer ache, my brain is sharper, and my sex life is better than ever."

You, too, can get all the benefits of exercise without torturing yourself. You can, in fact, get *more* benefit from the type of exercise you enjoy enough to make it a part of your way of life.

BUILD LIFESAVING
HDL WITH EXERCISE

It has been known for a long time that regular exercise would help prevent heart disease by lowering the amount of cholesterol and triglycerides in the blood. It was not discovered until recently, however, that regular exercise can stimulate the production of a cholesterol carrier that will actually *protect* the arteries! We now know that cholesterol is transported through the arteries by small particles of fat and protein called lipoproteins. *Low*-density lipoproteins deposit cholesterol in arterial walls. *High*-density lipoproteins carry cholesterol to the liver where the cholesterol is converted to bile and excreted by the gall bladder. Exercise increases the amount of high-density lipoproteins in your blood!

So, in addition to reducing your body weight and strengthening your heart, exercise helps your body get rid of excess cholesterol by providing it with transportation to disposal centers.

You can further aid the formation of high-density lipoproteins by taking Vitamin C and lecithin and by cutting down on the fats and sugars in your diet, substituting a small amount of vegetable oil. An increased amount of *fiber* in your diet helps lower blood cholesterol by stimulating the excretion of bile from your gall bladder. The type of diet recommended in Chapter 1 will supply the nutrients, the fatty acids, and the fiber your body needs to prevent a build-up of cholesterol and low-density lipoprotein in your blood.

Now you can see why both diet and exercise are such important parts of the *Peter Lupus Body-Improvement Program.*

The Cases of Clyde and James

Clyde A. discovered during a routine medical checkup that his blood cholesterol was up to a dangerous level of 600 milligrams percent (per 100 milliliters of blood)—far above the normal of 150 to 300 milligrams. (For the best of health, blood cholesterol should not go above 180 milligrams percent.) Since Clyde was also overweight, he was instructed to follow the 10 basic rules outlined in Chapter 1 and to begin walking and jogging. In less than six months, both his weight and his cholesterol were down to normal. "I'm happy to lose all that excess fat," Clyde reported, "but I'm even more pleased that my cholesterol is down. I didn't mind so much being fat, but I certainly did not want to die of a heart attack."

Triglycerides (blood fats) are also often elevated—and they can be just as dangerous as excess cholesterol. James H. had a normal blood cholesterol of 240 milligrams percent, but his triglyceride level was up to a whopping 800 milligrams percent! (Triglycerides should not go above 150 milligrams.) James got his triglycerides down simply by playing tennis and eliminating sugar and white-flour products from his diet. "Your program probably saved my life," Jack told us. "I'd recommend it for anyone."

Exercise is just as important as diet in reducing high blood levels of cholesterol and triglycerides. In fact, in some cases, exercise alone will do the job.

There are, of course, many other good reasons why you should exercise regularly.

MUSCLES AID YOUR HEART
IN PUMPING BLOOD

We have all seen persons faint from standing still too long. The reason this happens is that when muscles aren't contracting they aren't helping the heart muscle pump blood. Without the aid offered by contraction of your skeletal muscles, your heart is barely able to pump blood through your body—especially to your brain when you are standing erect. Your muscles actually serve as subsidiary pumps, and the older you become the more important it is to exercise your muscles. Tests show that blood flow through the muscles of the average 35-year-old American is 60 percent less than in younger persons. The reason for this, in part, is lack of exercise. And the less the muscles are exercised the greater the load placed on the heart. We are sad to note that most American men are in such poor physical condition that they are middle-aged at 26 years of age!

Poor circulation after middle age can result in a variety of disorders ranging from inability to think clearly to loss of a leg. Persons who sit day after day without exercising often develop blood clots in leg veins that have been distended and inflamed by pooling of blood. Obviously, regular exercise is essential for good health and a long life, but it need not be strenuous or punishing.

Leg Exercise Is the Most Important

Next to your heart, the muscles of your legs are the most important "blood pumps" in your body. You can activate these pumps simply by walking. When you set up your body-improvement program, try to include a recreational activity such as bicycling, tennis, or golf that requires you to use your legs. Swimming greatly aids circulation.

Buster Crabbe, a 1932 gold medal winner in Olympic swimming, best known for his "Flash Gordon" movie series, keeps fit by swimming. At the age of 70, he swims an average of 2,000 yards a day. He still has a 45-inch chest and a 34-inch waist at a body weight of 180 pounds—and he still looks like Flash Gordon.

"Swimming is the best exercise," Crabbe insists, "especially for older people, because the body is weightless in water. It takes the stress off joints. As we get older, many of us develop calcium deposits, bursitis, or arthritis, particularly in the lower back. Their effects can be relieved by exercising in water."

When comedian *Scatman Crothers* isn't working in a movie or on TV, he usually keeps active by playing golf or strumming his guitar. "Combining golf and dancing gives me all the exercise I need," he says.

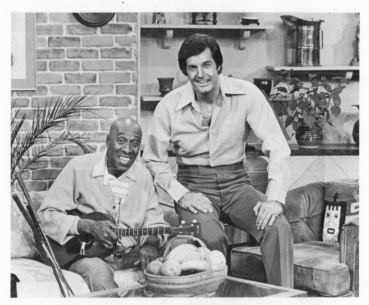

Scatman Crothers of TV's "Chico and the Man" gets plenty of walking exercise by playing golf regularly.

Paul Newman also swims for exercise. "I swim, day in, day out, no matter what the weather," he says.

Bob Hope is still fit, active, and hard at work at 74 years of age. He makes hundreds of public appearances each year. "I couldn't do it if I didn't exercise," he maintains. "I play a lot of golf, take long walks— at least two miles at night after my shows, and I watch my diet."

While Bob Hope is walking at night, *Pat Boone* is jogging. "I'm a night jogger," Boone says. "I run at least two miles every night, and more if I have the time."

Undoubtedly, the circulatory stimulation these entertainers get from their exercise helps to keep them youthful and fit. Regular exercise will help you, too.

Follow actress *Dody Goodman's* example and do something each day that requires full contraction of your thigh muscles. In her new role on the "Mary Tyler Moore Hour," Dody is just as funny and vivacious as she was on the "Mary Hartman" show.

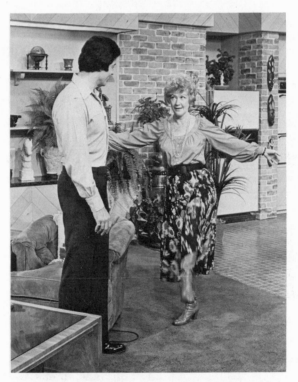

TV actress Dody Goodman of "Mary Hartman, Mary Hartman" stimulates her circulation daily by doing leg exercises in her home.

Well-Toned Muscles
Burn Calories 24 Hours a Day!

The number of calories burned by the body in an exercise program is usually measured during the actual performance of the exercise. There is now some evidence to indicate, however, that when muscles are exercised regularly they dispose of excess calories in metabolic fires that burn *24 hours a day.* It seems that the metabolic activity in muscles, in maintaining and repairing muscle fibers, requires a considerable number of calories while you are resting—while your body is in a basal metabolic state. Furthermore, when your diet is made up of fresh, natural foods, and you use your muscles as nature intended, your metabolic processes and the appetite mechanism in your brain will automatically balance your appetite and your caloric needs.

We all know active people who seem to be able to eat anything they want without gaining weight. Their bodies may be disposing of excess calories by burning them in well-toned muscle fibers that literally hum with chemical activity.

So, to repeat our earlier advice, you should exercise regularly so that you can eat generously to get the nutrients you need to look good and feel good, even if you aren't overweight.

MEASURE YOUR FITNESS
WITH YOUR PULSE RATE

If you are beginning exercise for the first time, you'll have to start out lightly to make sure that you don't place too much strain on your heart and your muscles. You can measure your fitness and your ability to perform work by counting your pulse before and after exercise.

Normally, a man's pulse should beat about 72 times a minute, a woman's about 75 times a minute. The more physically unfit you are the higher your pulse will be. A resting pulse rate higher than 80 beats a minute, for example, is usually an indication of poor fitness. *If your resting pulse rate is over 92, your chances of dying young are four times greater than if you had a resting pulse lower than 67.* But don't despair. As you become better conditioned by regular exercise, your pulse rate will become lower, indicating improved fitness and a stronger, more efficient heart.

You can avoid overexertion by exercising only as much as necessary to get your pulse rate up to 120 during the actual performance of the exercise. Of course, as you become more fit it will take more and more exercise to get your pulse rate up to 120—and your resting pulse will become lower and lower.

How to Record Your Pulse

Before you begin your exercise program, record your resting pulse rate while sitting and while standing. Normally, your standing pulse will be a little higher than your sitting pulse. If your standing pulse is 20 or more beats higher than your sitting pulse, however, this is another sign of poor physical fitness and may warrant a heart examination by a doctor.

Your pulse rate will be higher after exercising, after eating, after smoking a cigarette, after drinking coffee, or when you are nervous or excited. The best time to check your pulse is in the morning before eating and before shouldering your daily responsibilities.

You can locate your pulse by placing the fingertips of your right hand over the inside of you left wrist at the base of your thumb. With a little practice, you can count your pulse for 30 seconds or for 60 seconds while watching the second hand on a watch. If you count for 30 seconds, be sure to double the count for the total number of beats per minute.

When you record your pulse immediately after exercising, you may be able to get a more accurate evaluation of your fitness by counting your pulse for six seconds and then adding a zero or multiplying by 10. The amount of stress placed on the heart is most evident during the first 15 seconds following an exertion—before your pulse rate has a chance to subside.

Your pulse rate should be back to normal after about five minutes of rest. If you haven't fully recovered after 10 minutes, see your doctor for a checkup.

Whatever method of counting you use to record your pulse rate, whether for six seconds or for one minute following an exertion, use the same method each time so that you can accurately evaluate your progress. And be sure to keep a record of your resting pulse rate.

Clarence E., a 54-year-old postal clerk, had a resting pulse rate of 96 when he started exercising under our guidance. After only eight weeks of regular exercise, his resting pulse was down to 76. "I feel 100 percent better," Clarence testified. "I have a lot more endurance and much more energy. I don't give out anymore when I perform routine chores. I've especially noticed that my heart does not pound like it used to when I exert myself or when I jump to answer my telephone."

CHOOSING A METHOD OF EXERCISE

There are many ways to exercise. You may do whatever suits you best. When we featured *Dinah Shore* in one of our previous books (*Peter Lupus' Guide to Radiant Health and Beauty*), we learned that she did not like to exercise for the sake of exercise. She preferred to get her exercise by participating in such sports as golf and tennis. So do a number of other fit and famous celebrities. *Farrah Fawcett* and *Mary Tyler Moore*, for example, play tennis. *Angie Dickinson* jogs and swims. *Carol Burnett* and *Ali MacGraw* exercise by dancing. *Kate Jackson* roller skates. *Marie Osmond* prefers outdoor activities—and she shares Dinah Shore's views. "I'm an outdoors person," Marie says. "I love to horseback ride and to play golf and tennis. But I hate to exercise for the sake of exercise."

TV actor *Harrison Page,* who starred in "Super-train," prefers to play tennis for exercise, but he includes other forms of exercise, such as sit-ups, for overall body strength and symmetry.

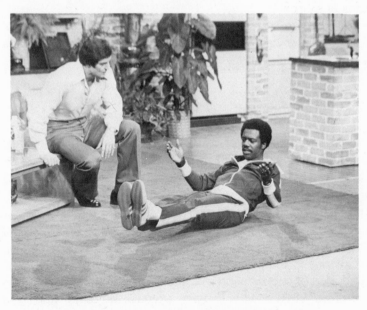

Harrison Page, co-star of the "CPO Sharkey" television series, combines tennis and calisthenics in a daily exercise program.

Actor *Anthony Quinn* gets recreational exercise by bicycling. "I've been cycling about six years," says Quinn, who is writing a book about bicycling. "I have about 12 bikes in cities around the world. I keep one in New York, one in Los Angeles, and so forth, so I don't have any problems when I go to a town."

Kirk Douglas also rides a bicycle for exercise. He can often be seen bicycling in the morning near his Beverly Hills home.

Dr. Joyce Brothers, a psychologist who often appears on television, prefers rope jumping. "I used to try to get my exercise by swimming in the hotel pool," she said. "But that ruined my hairdo and meant I had to spend time at the hair dresser. Now, I take my jump rope with me and exercise in my room."

Actress *Ann-Margret* also jumps rope. "I can jump rope for 10 minutes," she claims with pride.

Most of us prefer recreational exercise. And judging from the physical appearance of celebrities who participate in sports for exercise, recreational activity is just as good or better than regimented calisthenics. So if you prefer to dance, swim, play tennis, or whatever, you can do so. Just do it regularly, at least every other day, for several minutes at a time.

Joanne Woodward takes a ballet lesson every day in order to stay fit. "Ballet dancers are as fit as any athlete," she maintains. Joanne also runs three miles a day!

Warming Up Is Important

No matter what type of exercise you do, even if it's ballet dancing, you should always warm up for the exercise by doing the exercise lightly for a few minutes before making a maximum effort. This will help protect your muscles from strain. Also, to prevent injury, you should always stop doing an exercise when you begin to experience distress or discomfort. You cannot become strong and fit overnight, so don't be in a hurry.

Exercise to the point of *moderate* fatigue. When you are overly fatigued, loss of coordination may result in an injury. Be guided by the way you feel. When you begin a new exercise, do only a small amount of the the exercise and then gradually do a little more each day. This way, using the day-after as a guide, you can avoid injury or sore muscles caused by overexertion.

Note: You can't strain a healthy heart. But if you have an undetected heart condition, you can protect your heart by increasing the amount of exercise you do slowly and progressively, always stopping at the point of distress.

Carol Burnett's look-alike co-star, talented *Vickie Lawrence,* has extended her endurance for singing, dancing, and slapstick comedy by exercising progressively at home. She starts lightly before beginning more strenuous movements.

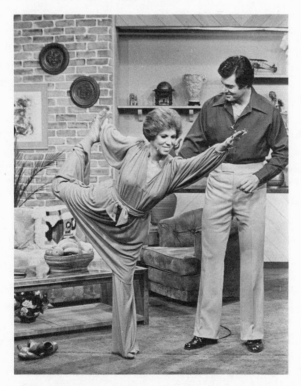

Vickie Lawrence of the "Carol Burnett Show" warms up by doing stretching exercises before dancing or exercising.

Moderation Is Best

Unless you have plenty of time for an exercise program, don't try to maintain a high level of fitness. *You can maintain a moderate level of fitness with only a fraction of the time and effort required to maintain maximum fitness.* Besides, if your work or social schedule forces you to occasionally discontinue your exercise for several days at a time, you'd find it impossible to maintain a high level of fitness. Furthermore, an attempt to do so on an irregular basis would result in injury. So be sensible. Don't go on a heavy program that you cannot follow consistently. It would be better to be moderate on a long-range program than to hurt yourself with an occasional heavy effort.

Walking, Jogging, and Roving

If you enjoy walking, you might be able to get all the calorie-burning, heart-stimulating exercise you need simply by taking long, brisk walks or by roving the neighborhood. All you have to do is begin by walking a block or two at a comfortable pace and then gradually increase the speed and distance over a period of several weeks. When you feel that brisk walking no longer offers you adequate exercise, you can begin combining walking and jogging. You simply jog until you are comfortably fatigued and then walk until you feel comfortably recovered before you begin to jog again.

Walking and jogging regularly, at least every other day for six weeks or longer, will reward you with a level of fitness that you can easily maintain. A record of your pulse rate should show considerable improvement in your physical fitness.

Nanette Fabray reduced her body weight and prepared herself physically for a special stage play by alternatively walking and running two miles up and down a hill every day. "I was winded at first," she admitted, "and I had to stop often, but it gave me so much more energy—and I went from a size eleven dress to a size eight!"

Lee Meriwether jogs by the clock—15 minutes at a time four or five times a week. When she discussed her jogging program on "Peter Lupus' Body Shop" television show, she shared the show with *Eula Weaver,* an 88-year-old jogger!

Is all this exercise worth the effort? Most actors think so. In fact, they consider it essential to exercise. "I don't think anything is harder work than making a movie," says *Kirk Douglas.* "If you're not physically fit, film making is difficult. If you don't have health and vitality, no matter what field you're in, you can't function."

Life itself is a stage, and if you're not physically fit you won't survive.

WHAT ABOUT SPOT REDUCING?

"But all I want to do is reduce my waist," argued Rosemary. "Why should I do anything but sit-ups?"

Sit-ups are fine, and everyone should do them to strengthen their abdominal muscles. But if it's *fat* you're trying to get rid of, you may be able to do it faster with some other form of exercise.

Any kind of exercise that burns calories will burn fat from all portions of your body—wherever fat is stored. Tennis, jogging, bicycling, and other activities that require use of the big muscles of your thighs may be more effective than sit-ups and other abdominal exercises in reducing your waistline. There is no such thing as "spot reducing." No matter where your body stores its fat, it will draw upon these stores when you burn more calories than you take in. *The best reducing exercise is the one that burns the most calories, and this usually means using your legs.*

HOW TO MAKE YOUR BODY
LOOK BETTER OVERALL

Jogging and brisk walking are great for burning calories and strengthening your heart, but they won't do much to strengthen your muscles in the upper portion of your body. Take your abdomen, for example. Even if you aren't fat, weak abdominal muscles may allow a pot belly or a hernia to develop, no matter how much you walk. If the muscles around your chest, upper back, and shoulders are under developed, you may be too weak to perform routine chores comfortably and you may be too bony-looking to be physically attractive. So even if you do walk or jog to keep your weight down, you should include a few upper body exercises to improve your overall physical appearance.

There are four or five basic exercises that anyone can do safely and effectively without danger of straining muscles and joints. Try to include them in your body-improvement program.

When cover model *Cheryl Tiegs* was asked what she does to maintain her beautiful body, she replied, "I exercise the hell out of it!" Cheryl's program calls for many of the same exercises described in this chapter. "I exercise in the gym three times a week for two hours each time," she said. "I work where I need it most by doing sit-ups, leg raises, and push-ups. I also play tennis three or four times a week."

Senator William Proxmire does 200 push-ups and 100 leg raises every morning before he runs five miles to his Washington office!

Shape Your Abdomen for a Trim Waistline

Simple sit-ups are best for strengthening the abdominal muscles. They must be done correctly, however, to be effective. If you are too weak to do sit-ups, do the trunk curl and the chair leg lift for a few weeks before you begin doing sit-ups regularly.

Trunk curl: Lie on your back on the floor (with your hands behind your head) and curl only your head and shoulders up from the floor. Concentrate on contracting your abdominal muscles during each curl. Repeat until your abdominal muscles tire. Try to do at least 12 repetitions. (See the photo.)

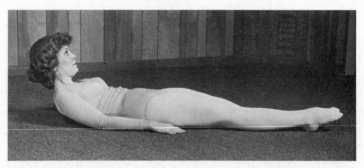

The trunk curl is a specific exercise for the abdominal muscles.

Chair Leg Lift: Many people cannot do sit-ups because they have weak hip flexors. This exercise will strengthen you hip flexors as well as tone your abdominal muscles.

Sit on the edge of a straight-back chair, lean back, and grasp each side of the chair seat with your hands. Starting with your legs locked out straight and your heels on the floor, lift your knees up toward your chest by bending your knees and your hips. Return to starting position and repeat at least 12 times. (See the photo.)

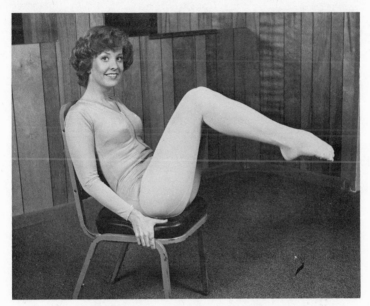

*Model Kim Ashbrook exercises her abdominal muscles
and hip flexors by doing chair leg lifts.*

Bent-knee sit-ups: When you are able to do more than 12 bent-knee sit-ups you don't have to do trunk curls and leg lifts unless you simply want to do some additional exercise to burn calories. The bent-knee sit-up alone will provide adequate exercise for your abdominal muscles and your hip flexors.

Lie on your back with your hands behind your head and your knees bent. Sit-up and touch your elbows to your knees. Be sure to *curl* your head and shoulders up from the floor when beginning the sit-up. (See the photo.)

Note: If you're top heavy and you find it difficult to do a sit-up, anchor your feet under the edge of a heavy sofa. This will shift some of the load from your abdominal muscles to your hip flexors, making the sit-up easier to do. Be sure to keep your knees bent, however, to reduce the leverage on your lower back.

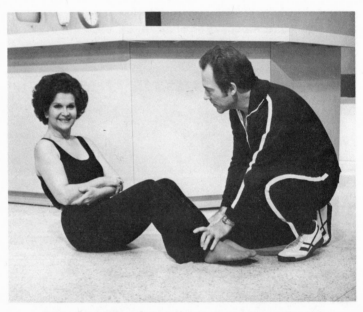

*TV hostess Helen Schuh demonstrates her method of
doing bent-knee sit-ups for a trim waistline.*

Warning: You should never do sit-ups with your legs locked out straight, whether your feet are anchored or not. Straight-leg sit-ups place too much strain on your lower spine and may result in back trouble. Besides, making the exercise more difficult by locking your legs out straight will simply reduce its effectiveness as an abdominal exercise.

Don't Strain!

In sit-ups, as in most exercises, it's best to relax your muscles momentarily between repetitions. This will allow a fresh flow of blood to remove accumulated waste products and prevent premature fatigue. When returning to the floor after performing a sit-up, for example, lie flat for a second or two before curling back up into a sit-up. Otherwise, blocking of the circulation by a sustained isometric contraction will limit the number of calories you burn by resulting in premature fatigue.

Richard Jaeckel, one of Hollywood's busiest and most talented actors, does sit-ups every day in order to stay fit for strenuous roles. His example encourages many Hollywood observers who pursue a physical training program.

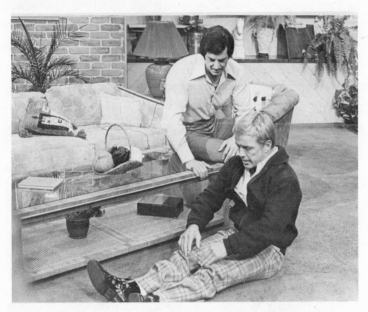

Movie and TV actor Richard Jaeckel stretches his hamstrings for increased flexibility by straightening his legs following a sit-up.

Fill Out Your Chest, Shoulders, and Arms

You don't need to do a large number of difficult and complicated exercises to develop the basic muscle groups of your body. A couple of simple exercises will do the job. Push-ups, and pull-ups, for example, will cover *all* the muscles of your upper body.

Modified push-up: If you're not accustomed to doing push-ups, or if you're not very strong, you should begin by doing *modified* push-ups. Just lie face down and push up from the floor, supporting your weight on your hands and knees. Work your way up to at least 10 repetitions. (See the photo.)

Regular push-ups: When you develop enough strength to do regular push-ups, you may simply switch from modified push-ups to regular push-ups. All you have to do is keep your body rigid during the push-up so that your weight is supported on your hands and your toes, as you see former "Laugh-In" star *Arte Johnson* doing. Arte, who hosts the TV game show· "Knockout," is literally a knockout doing push-ups. He does them regularly to maintain upper body strength.

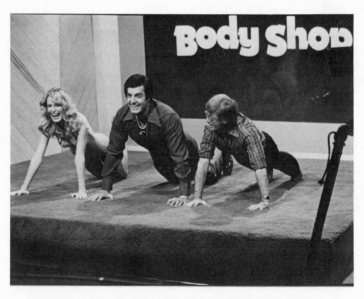

Comedian Arte Johnson demonstrates a regular push-up while Peter Lupus and actress Taaffe O'Connell do a less difficult modified *push-up.*

Modified pull-ups: Very few people can chin the bar in sufficient repetitions to be beneficial. Here, again, the exercise may be modified to permit comfortable performance of the exercise.

Arm-waving calisthenics are great for toning muscles, but they don't develop the reserve strength you need to make good use of your body. Furthermore, light calisthenics won't thicken your muscles enough to give your body pleasing contours. So if you want the best-looking body possible, you should do exercises that are resistant enough to prevent you from doing more than 12 to 15 repetitions.

To do a modified pull-up, place two arm chairs about two feet apart. Place a mop handle across the arms of the chairs. Lie down between the chairs and reach up so that you can grasp the mop handle with both hands. Pull your chest up to the handle, keeping your body rigid and your heels on the floor. Work your way up to at least 10 repetitions. (See the photo.)

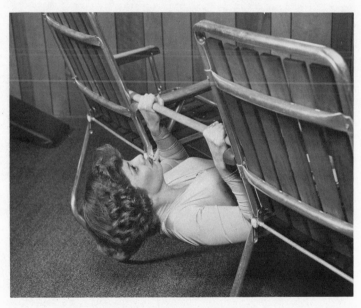

*The modified pull-up is a great arm and back exercise for
women as well as for men.*

Mold Your Thighs and Hips with Squats

If your thighs are thin and underdeveloped, you should do squatting exercises. Running may not enlarge your thigh muscles enough to give them a pleasing appearance.

Flat-footed squat: Hold onto a bed post for balance—and for assistance if necessary—and squat. Keep you head up and your spine as vertical as possible. Try to keep both feet flat on the floor while squatting. This will assure more all-around development of the muscles in your hips and thighs. If you have difficulty squatting flat-footed, place a board under your heels. Work your way up to 12 to 15 repetitions. (See the photo.)

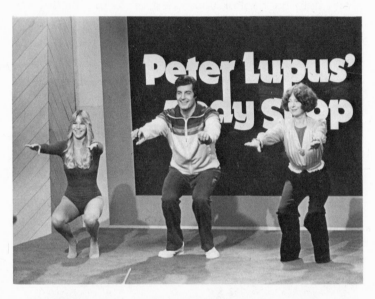

Model Sandy Serrano (left) is squatting on her toes to shape her thighs while physical fitness instructor Judith Stransky (right) demonstrates a hip-shaping flat-footed squat.

Graduate to Barbell Exercises

When your body fat has been reduced and your muscles have been strengthened by recreational activities and basic exercise, take a good look at yourself in a mirror. Are you as muscular as you want to be? Does your body have pleasing contours? Are some portions of your body too small or too bony?

You can change the shape of your body, or you can increase the size of any portion of your body, with the barbell exercises described in the next chapter. *Underweight men and women who have trouble gaining weight will find barbell exercises especially effective for adding lean tissue.*

So if you want a body that's strong as well as attractive, take the next step and try our barbell exercises.

SUMMARY

1. You must exercise at least twice a week for exercise to be safe and effective.

2. You can burn more calories with frequent abbreviated workouts than with one long marathon program.

3. To strengthen your heart muscle, you should exercise vigorously enough to maintain a pulse rate of about 120 beats per minute for several minutes.

4. You can maintain a moderate degree of fitness with only a fraction of the time required to maintain peak physical fitness.

5. Regular exercise will protect your heart and blood vessels by *lowering* the amount of cholesterol and triglycerides in your blood while *increasing* the formation of high-density lipoproteins.

6. Using the big muscles of your thighs will aid the circulation of blood as well as burn a maximum number of calories.

7. As you become more fit, your pulse rate will become lower.

8. Remember that it takes at least six weeks of regular exercise to acquire a moderate level of fitness.

9. If you want to improve the *appearance* of your body, you should include a few basic exercises to develop the major muscle groups.

10. If you have a thin, bony body, you can increase the size of your muscles by doing the barbell exercises described in Chapter 3.

3

How Movie and TV Actors Build and Shape Their Bodies For Demanding Roles

Most women are surprised to learn that lifting weights will make them more shapely. Exercising with barbells and dumbbells is usually thought of as a joint-straining form of exercise reserved solely for men. The truth is, however, that a woman can benefit just as much as a man in a properly designed weight-training program.

When a man lifts weights in a progressive resistance exercise program, there is a rapid increase in the size and strength of his muscles. It's possible for a man to develop his muscles until they are literally *huge*—if that's what he wants. A woman, however, while she can enlarge her muscles to some extent, cannot develop muscles like a man. Female hormones *prevent* the development of huge, sinewy muscles. But a woman *can* develop her muscles to improve her physical appearance. And in bony areas of the body, she can develop muscular padding that will add greatly to the beauty and symmetry of her figure.

Actress *Jamie Lee Curtis* learned from her father *Tony Curtis* that resistive exercise is just as beneficial for women as for men. She exercises regularly to maintain her physical strength and development.

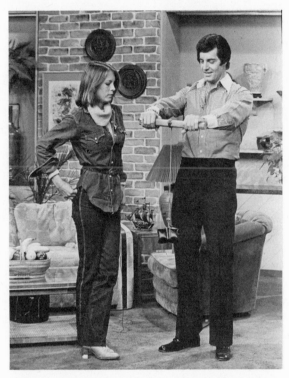

Jamie Lee Curtis of television's "Operation Petticoat" instructs Peter Lupus in how to use a wrist roller, her favorite arm and shoulder exercise device.

Actually, without well-developed muscles to mold the fatty tissue that normally covers the female body, a woman cannot have a truly beautiful body. Practically all of the present-day bathing suit beauties lift weights to develop their skeletal muscles. Female athletes are also lifting weights to improve their athletic abilities. Tennis star *Billie Jean King*, for example, lifts weights regularly. So does Olympic swimmer *Shirley Babashoff.* At Tennessee State University, the entire women's track team lifts weights!

Kathy Schmidt, a U.S. record holder in the javelin throw, lifts weights primarily to improve her athletic ability, but she also *enjoys* lifting. "I love to lift," she says. "It makes me feel good to do it. I feel healthier, stronger, and I can see my body taking a different shape. It's also a great release from aggressions." (*Broken Patterns,* Dodd, Mead and Company, 1977.)

Singer *Trini Lopez* lifts weights to improve her health. "I do my health a good turn by lifting weights regularly," she said when describing her health program.

Every woman, even if she is healthy, can use some additional strength. Chores are easier to perform and the days are less fatiguing when muscles are strong. Best of all, from a standpoint of beauty, *muscle-building exercises will do more for a woman's body than any other single measure.*

The case of Marcella A. is typical of the women who have benefited from the weight-training portion of the *Peter Lupus Body-Improvement Program.* When she first began weight training, her calves were too small, her thighs widely spaced, her shoulders too bony, and her hips were flabby. It took only three months of exercise for Marcella to enlarge her calves, firm up her body, and fill in deficient areas. "I literally changed the shape of my body," she reported with amazement. "For the first time in my life, I feel that I look pretty good in a bathing suit. I wish I had started weight training 10 years ago."

Weight training can produce even more dramatic changes in the physical appearance of men.

BUILD MUSCLES RAPIDLY
WITH WEIGHT TRAINING

When steel-helmeted, iron-masked *Darth Vadar* appeared on the screen in the movie "Star Wars," the evil power he radiated sent chills up and down the spines of the movie audience. The "evil" was simply an effect produced by sound effects and costuming, but the power was real. Underneath that formidable costume was *David Prouse,* a six-foot-six former British Olympic heavyweight weight-lifting champion who maintains his size and strength by lifting weights. Prouse first began lifting weights at 14 years of age, after spending 10 months in bed with a mysterious disease that doctors said would cripple him

With the arrival of *Arnold Schwarzenegger* on the movie screen, muscles are definitely "in." This former "Mr. Universe" and "Mr. Olympia" is now in great demand as an actor and has even replaced thinner males as a sex symbol. When Schwarzenegger appeared in the centerfold of *Cosmopolitan* magazine, he was an instant favorite.

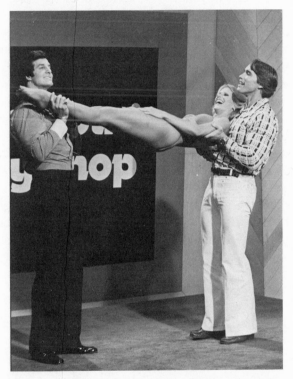

Peter Lupus and Arnold Schwarzenegger, star of the movie "Stay Hungry," demonstrate resistive isotonic exercise by lifting actress Shannon Wilcox.

for life. "I ignored the pessimism of the doctors," he stated, "and launched myself on an exercise and weight-lifting program."

Today, David Prouse is a successful actor whose powerful physique earns him many special and unique movie roles. When other actors need to build and shape their bodies for a demanding role, Prouse often lends a helping hand. When *Christopher Reeve* was cast in the movie role of "Superman," for example, Prouse spent six weeks getting him into shape with barbell exercises. Reeve added 30 pounds of weight to his six-foot, four-inch frame! He was such a hit as Superman that plans are already underway for the filming of "Superman II." His latest movie, "Somewhere in Time," features talent rather than muscles.

Lou Ferrigno, a former "Mr. Universe" who portrays The Hulk in the television series "The Incredible Hulk," maintains his 275 pounds of muscular body weight by lifting weights daily.

Many actors, such as *Sylvester Stallone,* lift weights to shape their bodies for special roles. When Stallone portrayed a boxer in the movie "Rocky," his massive physique added a touch of realism that could not be faked in movie making. And his physical appearance was so appealing to movie goers that he soon became a poster favorite among young people.

If you want to build and strengthen your body as rapidly as possible for a special role in life, to improve your athletic ability, or simply to improve your physical appearance, you can do so by lifting weights. If your body is thin and weak, a few basic barbell exercises performed every other day for several weeks will do more for your physical appearance than years of calisthenics.

STRONG MUSCLES MAKE LIFE EASIER!

Both men and women can do the same basic barbell exercises. The only difference is that women won't use as much weight or do as many sets as a man who is striving for maximum muscular development. If an exercise calls for eight repetitions, for example, the individual simply adds enough weight to the bar to permit comfortable performance of the exercise. Since a man develops size and strength much faster than a woman, he will automatically use more weight than a woman.

Basically, then, all you have to do, whether you are a man or a woman, is to select a comfortable amount of weight for each exercise each time you work out and let your muscles take care of themselves. As you become stronger, you'll progressively increase the amount of weight you use in each exercise. If you are a man, your muscles will soon begin to bulge and ripple with new size and strength. If you are a woman, development of your muscles will fill in deficient areas and give your body the full, firm contours that you need to be physically beautiful. And with an increase in strength, you'll finish each day with strength and energy to spare!

Ricardo Montalban, who has developed a fine physique lifting weights, first started exercising after injuring his back while filming a movie. "The accident left me with a partial paralysis of the leg," he recalled, "and I knew that if I let the leg muscles atrophy I might never walk again. I began exercising and have never stopped. I need to be in good shape for the physical and sometimes seemingly impossible demands made on me by Hollywood."

Tony Randall, one of Hollywood's hardest working stars, lifts weights regularly to maintain the strength and endurance he needs to withstand the strain of his schedule.

Everyday life places seemingly impossible demands on many of us. We can all use some additional strength in meeting these demands. Lifting weights is the best and easiest way to build and maintain the extra strength we need.

The Case of Arthur D.

Arthur D. is an insurance salesman who spends long hours collecting debits and selling insurance. "I'm exhausted at the end of the day," he complained. "I just don't feel like doing anything."

Since Arthur's body was weak and flabby, we started him on weight training. He did four basic exercises every other day for several weeks before reporting back to us. "I feel great," he reported with obvious enthusiasm. "I'm not nearly so tired at the end of the day. My physique has improved so much that I want to continue with weight training."

Most men, like Arthur, become completely sold on weight training when they experience the resulting increase in size and strength. This is why so many bodybuilders never give up weight training—they like the physical improvement that results from lifting weights.

Don't worry about building too much muscle, men. Just having large muscles does not mean that you'll become "muscle-bound."

The truth is that weight training will increase your speed and flexibility as you grow bigger and stronger. This is why most athletes, including swimmers, now lift weights. Besides, you don't have to build any more muscle than you want.

And don't worry about muscle turning to fat when you quit training. Muscles do not turn to fat; they simply *shrink* if you quit exercising. It takes only a small amount of exercise to maintain muscular development acquired by weight training. It's not likely that you'll ever quit exercising completely if you are health conscious.

HOW TO MAKE YOUR OWN WEIGHTS

Most sporting goods stores sell barbells and dumbbells. If you invest in a set of weights, buy the *iron* weights; they'll never wear out.

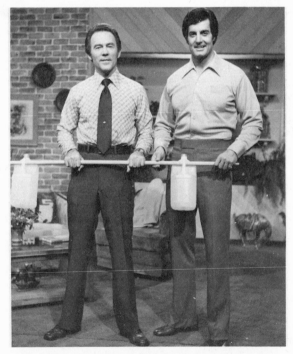

Dr. Samuel Homola and Peter Lupus demonstrate use of a homemade barbell made with plastic milk jugs and a mop handle.

The sand-filled plastic weights may be more trouble than they're worth, and they may eventually crack open.

If you don't have access to commercial weights, you can make your own. All you have to do is flatten the ends of a four-foot section of water pipe and then harden gallon cans of cement on each end of the pipe. If you really want to get fancy, you can slip a larger pipe over the smaller pipe (*before* attaching the cans of cement) so that the bar will have a rotating sleeve. Otherwise, you may have to use gloves so that the bar can rotate in your hands without causing blisters. Some industrious weightlifters make barbell "plates" by pouring concrete into molds containing chicken wire.

If you are a beginner in weight training, you won't need much weight. Women, for example, often start with only 25 or 30 pounds, and men with only about 50 pounds. This includes the weight of the bar, of course, when commercial barbells are used. The easiest way to make a homemade barbell (especially for ladies and children) is to fill plastic gallon containers with sand or water and then place one on each end of a pipe or mop handle. (The handle of a plastic gallon milk container will slip nicely over the end of a mop handle.) You can increase the weight in these containers by adding sand, water, wet sand, or lead shot. Begin with sand and then add water to the sand as you become stronger.

THE BASIC RULES OF WEIGHT TRAINING

After you have trained with weights for a while, you'll develop your own method of training. To begin with, however, you should follow certain basic rules. *Both men and women should follow these rules* until they become advanced enough and knowledgeable enough to alter these rules to suit their special needs.

Rule 1: Selecting a Weight

In each exercise you do, *select a weight that will allow you to perform the recommended number of repetitions without straining.*

For example, if an exercise calls for eight repetitions, you should be able to do 12 repetitions if you really had to. When you can do 12 repetitions without straining, you can add enough weight to the bar to again make the exercise sufficiently resistant in eight repetitions. You don't have to add weight to the bar at a predetermined rate. Be guided by the way you feel. As you become stronger, you'll automatically add the correct amount of weight.

Rule 2: Frequency of Workouts

If you are lifting weights to gain weight or to enlarge your muscles, *you should not work out more often than every other day.* Three times a week, on Monday, Wednesday, and Friday, with complete rest on Saturday and Sunday, is the most commonly used schedule.

In order for muscle fibers to grow, they must have adequate time between workouts to repair and rebuild. As your strength increases and the amount of weight you use increases, your muscle fibers will thicken in order to meet the demands of the work placed upon them. This is why weight training for the purpose of increasing strength or enlarging muscles is called "progressive resistance exercise."

Note: Muscle building increases the *thickness* rather than the number of muscle fibers. A "muscle man," for example, has the same number of muscle fibers he was born with. His muscle fibers have simply thickened as a result of taxing them with progressive resistance exercise.

Rule 3: Breathing During Barbell Exercises

No matter what you have learned about breathing during the performance of yoga and other forms of exercise, *you should always exhale when you are exerting yourself during the performance of a barbell exercise.* You should *never* hold your breath during any exercise. Try to breath rhythmically when you are exercising.

Holding your breath while exerting yourself will increase the pressure in your chest and abdomen and reduce the return flow of blood to your heart, resulting in lack of adequate blood flow to your brain. This could result in a blackout, which could be dangerous. So remember: Don't hold your breath!

Ron Masak, star of the movie "Harper Valley PTA," like many actors, lifts weights to thicken his muscles so that he'll look good when dressed. Without well-developed muscles, clothes do not fit properly. So even if you never wear a bathing suit, you should develop your muscles so that you'll look shapelier in clothes.

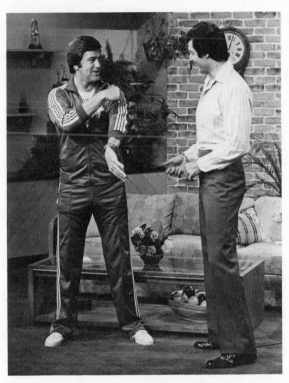

Ron Masak points out the triceps development he has acquired by lifting weights.

Rule 4: Eating to Build Muscles

Everyone should eat properly prepared foods in a balanced diet that supplies all the essential nutrients. If you are lifting weights to enlarge your muscles, however, you may need a little more protein than the average person.

Chicken, fish, lean meats, cheese, milk, and eggs are the best sources of high-quality protein. Seeds, soybeans, wheat germ, and nuts can supply additional protein in a balanced diet.

In your effort to gain weight, be careful not to add fat to your body by eating refined carbohydrates. All the carbohydrate in your diet should come from such *natural* foods as fruits, vegetables, and potatoes. Excess body fat is harmful to your health, and the foods that produce such fat contribute to the development of diabetes, heart disease, hardened arteries, and other diseases.

Try to balance your meals with the basic natural foods, and then include a little extra protein. Between-meal snacks of baked chicken or uncreamed cottage cheese, for example, will provide additional low-fat protein.

How Much Protein Do You Need?

It's generally believed that the average person needs about one gram of protein for each 2.2 pounds of bodyweight, or about 70 grams of protein a day. Unless you are actively engaged in muscle building, eating larger amounts of protein may only contribute extra calories. So don't eat just to be eating. Eat according to the amount of exercise you're doing and the size of your muscles. The more you exercise and the larger your muscles, the more protein you need. Some bodybuilders consume a few hundred grams of protein daily to assure that they get adequate protein for repair, growth, and maintenance of muscle fibers. Keep an eye on your body. If you begin to look fat, or if you can pinch up more than an inch of fat anywhere on your body, you're eating too much.

You can estimate the amount of protein you're consuming each day if you know how much protein you're getting from foods of animal origin. The average serving (about 3½ ounces) of meat, chicken, or fish supplies about 25 grams of protein. Once cup of skimmed milk or yogurt contains around 9 grams of protein, and one cup of cottage cheese about 38 grams of protein. Two eggs will supply from 11 to 14 grams of protein, depending upon the size of the eggs.

If you're not intolerant to milk, you can make a good high-protein drink by adding milk powder to milk. One cup of skimmed milk powder mixed into a quart of skimmed milk, for example, will provide a total of 65 grams of high-quality protein. If milk gives you indigestion, you can use protein powder made from fish, eggs, soybeans, and other sources of complete protein.

Remember that you can get protein from many different foods. Nuts, seeds, vegetables, and grains, for example, supply an incomplete protein that combines in your body to form a complete protein. So you don't have to get all your protein from foods of animal origin if you eat a variety of foods in a balanced diet.

Rule 5: Advancing with Sets

When you first begin doing barbell exercises, you do only one set of each exercise. For example, if the exercise calls for eight repetitions, you do eight consecutive repetitions and then go on to a different exercise. *As you become stronger and more muscular, you can begin doing two sets of each exercise,* using the first set as a warmup for the second set. This means that you first do the exercise with a fairly light weight in order to prepare yourself for the use of a heavier weight in a second set. This way, you can stimulate greater muscular growth by pumping blood through your muscles (hence the expression "pumping iron"). With a proper warmup, you can work up to the use of a heavier weight without hurting yourself.

Women may prefer to continue doing only one set of each exercise. But men who want exceptional size and strength should work up to two or more sets of each exercise over a period of several months.

Note: If you do more than one set of a barbell exercise, rest a minute or two between sets, until your muscles feel sufficiently recovered to go on to the next set. Don't rest so long, however, that you allow your muscles to "cool off." Remember that muscles must be warmed with an increased flow of blood to lift weights safely and effectively.

Basic Barbell Exercises
For Men and Women

All of the barbell exercises described in this chapter are designed

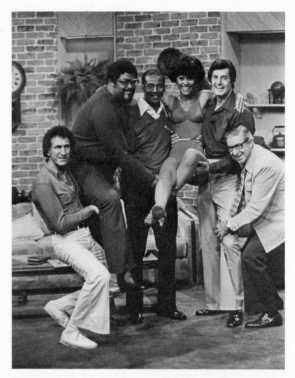

*Don Davis, Rosie Grier, Ernie Banks, Kellie Patterson,
Peter Lupus, and Bill Baldwin get isometric weight lifting
exercise by attempting to lift each other.*

for use by men and women who are *beginners* in weight training. This means that only *basic* exercises will be used to develop the major muscle groups. Once you become accustomed to lifting weights, you can include other more specialized exercises with barbells and dumbbells. In the meantime, stick with the exercises described in this chapter—and don't overdo it! If you like, you may do only the exercises you feel you need most.

Men can expect rapid muscular gains from weight training. Regular training for six weeks or longer can result in a gain of several pounds of muscle. Alvin D. gained 10 pounds of muscle during his first six weeks of training. "After only three months of lifting weights," Alvin testified, "I have gained a total of 15 pounds of solid muscle! Everyone is telling me that I look like Charles Atlas."

The best way to detect muscular gain is to measure your biceps, your chest, and your thighs. Record your measurements for future comparison. Now, let's get started.

Develop Your Chest with Bench Presses

The supine bench press is performed by lying on your back on a low bench and pressing a barbell from your chest straight up to arm's length. Use a shoulder-width grip on the bar, with the palms of your hands turned toward your feet. (See the photo.)

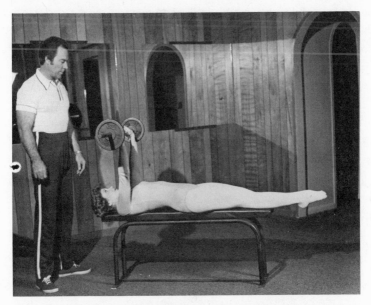

*Dr. Samuel Homola spots beauty queen Kim Ashbrook
during a chest-building bench press.*

To perform this exercise properly, you should press and lower the weight *smoothly* for at least eight repetitions. Exhale as you press the weight.

As you become stronger, you may begin to use such a heavy weight that you'll have to have someone place the weight on your chest while you're lying on the bench. Or you may purchase a special "bench-press bench" that has a supporting rack. You can find such a bench in most sporting goods stores.

The bench press will develop the triceps muscles on the back of your arms and the anterior deltoid muscles on the front of your shoulders as well as the pectoral muscles on the front of your chest.

Although the major pectoral muscles of the woman are hidden by overlying breast tissue, development of these muscles will help shape and enlarge the breasts.

Men and women who are so bony in the upper portion of their chest that their ribs are visible can pad this area by doing *inclined* bench presses. You can do this exercise on a special bench that inclines about 45 degrees, or you may simply lean back against an inclined board. Pressing a barbell while your body is supported on an incline will activate the *minor* pectoral muscles, which are located *above* the major pectoral muscles.

Pad Your Shoulders with Upright Rowing Motions

Nothing looks worse than bony shoulders. And when there is so little muscle on your shoulders that the bones protrude sharply, you'll be less appealing to the opposite sex—dressed or undressed. So developing your shoulder muscles will give you more sex appeal as well as improve your physical appearance.

Women do not need to worry about their shoulders getting too wide as a result of developing their muscles. Wide shoulders are the result of an inherited bone structure. Developing the shoulder muscles will simply provide the padding you needed to eliminate the sharp appearance of a bony shoulder girdle.

In any event, both men and women can benefit from shoulder exercises that develop the deltoid muscles. The most effective exercise for this purpose is the upright rowing motion with a barbell.

Stand erect while holding a barbell down at arm's length in front. Grip the bar palms down, with your hands about four inches apart. Lift the bar up to your neck, pointing your elbows forward and up. Lower the bar to starting position and repeat at least seven more times. (See the photo.)

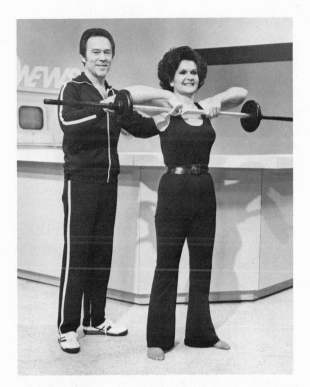

*Dr. Samuel Homola instructs actress Helen Schuh in the
performance of upright rowing motions for shoulder
development.*

Be careful not to use so much weight in this exercise that you must lean backward or jerk the weight up to complete a repetition.

Strengthen Your Arms with Curls

Whether you are a man or a woman, you must have a certain amount of arm strength to perform simple chores. So even if you don't feel that you need to develop the biceps muscle on the front of your upper arm, you should at least make sure that your arms aren't weak. The barbell curl is absolutely the best exercise you can do to develop and strengthen your biceps. There isn't a man alive who does not take pride in displaying a well-developed biceps—and this is why the barbell curl is so popular among men.

Stand erect while holding a barbell down at arm's length in front. Grip the bar palms up, with your hands about shoulder-width apart. Keep your elbows close to your sides and curl the bar up to your neck, exhaling as you curl. Return to starting position and repeat seven more times. Be careful not to use so much weight that you have to cheat in the performance of a curl. Remember that this exercise is designed strictly for your biceps. (See the photo.)

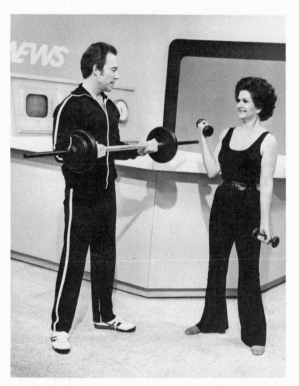

Barbell and dumbbell curls enlarge the biceps.

Strengthen Your Back
with Bent-Over Rowing Motions

Men will be especially interested in this exercise, since it builds the back muscles that give the upper body a "V" shape. It also strengthens back muscles that help protect the spine. It must be done *properly,* however, to avoid straining your back. *If you already have back trouble, don't do this exercise.* Instead, turn to Chapter 7 and do some of the exercises that are designed to strengthen your back without placing a strain on your spine.

To do a bent-over rowing motion, stand in front of a barbell that's resting on the floor. Bend forward by bending your hips and your knees and grip the barbell with a shoulder-width, palms-down grip. *Keep your head up and your back flat* and lift the barbell from the floor to your waist. Keep your arms close to your sides while touching the bar to your abdomen. (See the photo.)

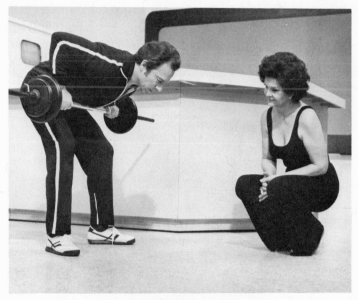

*Bent-over rowing motions, observed by Helen Schuh,
strengthen the back.*

Be careful not to use so much weight that you cannot do at least eight comfortable repetitions. Exhale while lifting the weight.

Shape and Develop Your Thighs and Hips with Squats

Can you squat all the way down and come back up without using your hands for assistance? If not, your thigh muscles are too weak to lift properly and to serve you adequately in an emergency.

Take off your clothes and take a look at yourself in a mirror. Are your thighs thin and flabby? Is there an unattractive space between your thighs? All of these problems are caused by lack of adequate muscular development. Without well-developed muscles, your thighs cannot possibly have the pleasing contours that make them physically appealing and sexually attractive.

Whether your thighs are weak or ugly, or both, you can shape and strengthen them with barbell squats. As you become stronger from squatting with a barbell, you can increase the size of your thighs and fill in deficient areas simply by adding a little more weight to your barbell.

You should *never strain* while squatting with a barbell. If you work your way up to the use of a fairly heavy weight, you might want to use a "squat rack" in your workouts. This is a frame that supports the

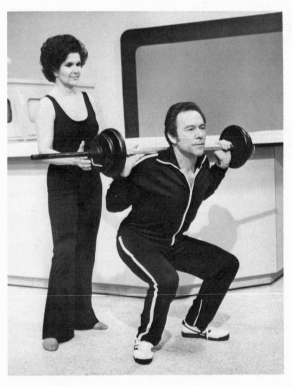

Barbell squats shape the hips and thighs.

barbell at shoulder level so that you can place and remove the bar from your shoulders simply by backing up to the rack.

To perform a barbell squat properly, keep your head up and your back as flat and as vertical as possible while squatting. A board under your heels may make it easier for you to maintain your balance. Be careful not to bounce at the bottom of the squat, lest you injure your knees or your back. Squat until your thighs and calves touch and then return to an erect position. Keep your squat under control by squatting slowly and smoothly. Do about eight repetitions. (See the photo.)

Expand Your Chest with Straight-Arm Pullovers

When you finish doing your squats, chances are you'll be breathing heavily. This is a good time to do a deep-breathing, chest-expanding exercise. Forced deep breathing when you don't need the oxygen can result in dizziness caused by "blowing off" carbon dioxide. So be sure to reserve your breathing exercises for a breathless period following squats or some other exercise that results in an oxygen debt.

The primary reason for doing straight-arm pullovers is to enlarge and deepen your rib cage. If you feel that your rib cage is already large enough and is symmetrical in appearance, you may choose not to do this exercise.

Lie on your back on the floor and hold a light weight at arm's length over your chest. A barbell bar or a five-pound dumbbell in each hand will be heavy enough. Lower the weight back over your head with straight arms (or with your elbows slightly bent), *inhaling deeply*

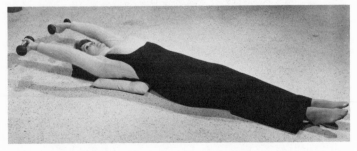

Straight-arm pullovers deepen the chest.

while the weight is being lowered to the floor. Concentrate on expanding and lifting your rib cage as high as you can. Exhale while returning to starting position. Repeat at least eight times. (See the photo.)

Note: You must use a *light* weight in this exercise so that your abdominal muscles won't contract and interfere with expansion of your rib cage. A small amount of weight will force the contraction of your pectoral muscles to lift your rib cage.

Enlarge Your Calves with Toe Rises

If you already have well-developed calves that are large enough to balance your physique or figure, you may not need to do a calf

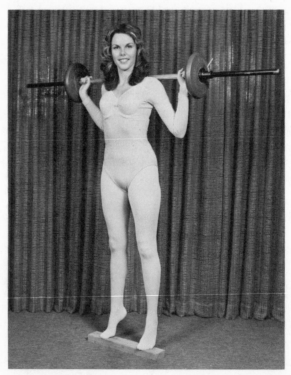

*Toe rises, demonstrated by model Jean Blackwell, enlarge
the calves.*

exercise. But if your calves are thin and weak, you can increase their size and strength—and improve their shape—by rising up and down on your toes while supporting a barbell.

Place a barbell across your shoulders behind your neck and rise up on your toes at least 15 times. A board under the forepart of your feet will make the exercise more effective by allowing you to drop your heels lower. (See the photo.)

Note: Since the calf muscles are denser than other body muscles, it's usually necessary to do 15 to 20 repetitions in toe rises (also called heel rises) to exercise the calves adequately.

What About Your Neck?

Most women won't be concerned about making their neck any larger. Men, however, who want to look as muscular and masculine as possible, might want to thicken their neck muscles. The easiest way to do this is to move your head against resistance applied by your hands.

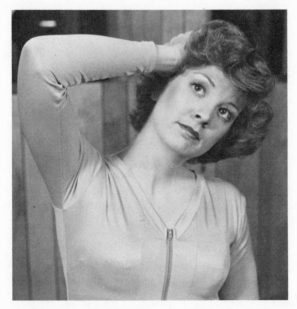

Kim Ashbrook demonstrates a resistive neck exercise that thickens neck muscles.

Just tilt your head forward, backward, and from side to side while resisting the movement with a hand placed against your head. Move your head against resistance in each direction for 12 to 15 repetitions or until your neck muscles tire. You'll be amazed at how fast your neck muscles respond to this simple exercise. (See the photo.)

EXTENDING YOUR PROGRAM

There are, of course, many other barbell exercises that you can do, such as the standing press, the shoulder shrug, and so on. But

John Grimek, the only man ever to win the AAU "Mr. America" title *twice*, used advanced methods of weight training to build his perfect physique. John's muscular development is unparalleled in the history of bodybuilding. He does many of the exercises described in this chapter.

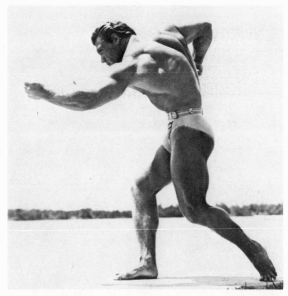

John Grimek, editor of Muscular Development *magazine, retired undefeated as the physique champion of the world after developing his muscles by lifting weights.*

unless you are an athlete pursuing an advanced form of training, or a bodybuilder training for physique competition, you do not need to do more than five or six exercises to cover all the major muscle groups of your body. To do more would simply overlap similar exercises and overload your body.

If you become advanced enough in your training to include more specialized barbell and dumbbell exercises, you can get additional instruction from such magazines as *Strength & Health* and *Muscular Development* or from your local spa. There isn't enough room in one chapter of a book to cover advanced weight training.

There is a great deal more to the *Peter Lupus Body-Improvement Program* than building large muscles. Good nutrition, care of your skin and hair, self help in the care of common ailments, and other aspects of developing and maintaining an attractive, healthy body are equally important. So be sure to read all the other chapters of this book. You'll learn in the next chapter how you can prevent the development of disease simply by making certain changes in your everyday health habits.

SUMMARY

1. Lifting weights is the best and easiest way to build and shape your body and fill in deficient areas.

2. Women as well as men can improve their physical appearance by lifting weights.

3. Female hormones and feminine fat prevent the development of overly large muscles in women.

4. Everyone can use some additional strength in performing chores and meeting emergencies.

5. Remember: In every barbell exercise you do, select a weight that will allow comfortable performance of at least eight repetitions.

6. You should never train more often than every other day with weights.

7. Always *exhale* when you are exerting yourself during a barbell exercise. Don't ever hold your breath!

8. In order to speed muscular development while lifting weights, include a little extra protein in a balanced diet of fresh, natural foods.

9. When you first begin weight training, you should do only five or six exercises to develop the major muscle groups.

10. Having an attractive body means having good teeth, skin, and hair as well as strong muscles, so be sure to study the remaining chapters of this book.

4

The Everyday Health Habits Of Stars at Home and at Work

According to a 1977 nutrition report released by a U.S. Senate Committee,* *six of the ten leading causes of death in the United States have been linked to our diet.* Too much fat, cholesterol, alcohol, sugar, and salt, for example, have been directly connected with heart disease, cancer, cerebrovascular disease (stroke), diabetes, arteriosclerosis, and cirrhosis of the liver.

We all know that smoking is a major cause of lung cancer. There is now some evidence to indicate that food additives and preservatives (substances not normally found in the body) can cause cancer. Excessive use of refined and processed foods that are deficient in fiber as well as nutrients also plays a role in the development of disease. Habitual use of processed foods not only fails to supply essential nutrients but also *drains* nutrients from the body.

---

*Dietary Goals for the United States, U.S. Government Printing Office, Washington, D.C. 20402.

Lack of adequate rest and exercise further weakens the body. If you are a "successful" person, chances are you're running yourself to death trying to keep up with the Joneses. This may place considerable nervous strain on your heart. Furthermore, the effects of stress may be contributing to a build-up of fat and other harmful substances in your blood. The Senate report on nutrition concluded that *food* we eat has more to do with the state of our health than any other single factor. What you learn in this chapter may be the most important part of your body-improvement program.

LENGTHEN YOUR LIFE
WITH GOOD HEALTH HABITS

Biochemist *Dr. Linus Pauling,* a two-time winner of the Nobel Prize, maintains that the average American could add from 16 to 24 years to his life simply by cutting down on sugar, refraining from smoking, and by taking optimum amounts of vitamins and minerals. Whatever the cause of disease, we know that few people die of old age. Biologists tell us that the human body should last at least 125 years! With a life span of only 75 years, the average person is killed by disease that destroys his body long before he lives out his allotted life span.

According to *Dr. Hans Selye,* the world's leading authority on stress, death is invariably caused by premature failure of an organ of the body. "In fact," he adds, "I do not think anyone has died of old age yet." Dr. Selye believes that we could enormously lengthen the average life span by living in better harmony with natural laws (*The Stress of Life,* McGraw-Hill).

Fortunately, almost all the leading causes of death are preventable. According to *Human Nutrition,* published by the U.S. Department of Agriculture (1971), "Most of the health problems underlying the leading causes of death in the United States could be modified by improvements in diet." And, like the Senate committee, they're talking about *food,* not cigarettes, alcohol, lack of exercise, and other factors that also contribute to bad health.

Obviously, there is *plenty* that you can do to improve your health and prolong your life. It's simply a matter of paying attention to your everyday health habits, with special attention to what you eat. The average American eats fat-rich meat three times a day, salts foods liberally, consumes up to 125 pounds of sugar a year, snacks on colas and hamburgers, fries his food in fat, eats refined carbohydrates, smokes cigarettes, drinks alcohol, and gets little or no exercise. It's no wonder that obesity, heart disease, and cancer are so common. Diabetes is presently the seventh most common cause of death, but projections indicate that the number of diabetics will *double* in the next 15 years!

You can take control of your life and change your health habits to *prevent* the development of many killer diseases. The celebrities who follow the *Peter Lupus Body-Improvement Program* are all instructed in the use of health measures that prolong life as well as improve physical appearance. With this book, we're offering you the same instructions—just as if we were talking to you personally.

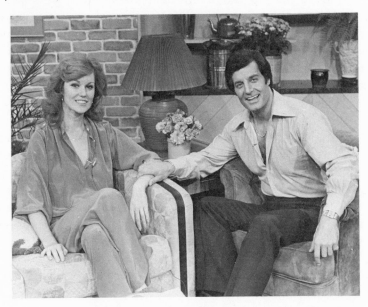

Barbara Rhodes, star of "Busting Loose," gets personal instruction from "Body Shop" host Peter Lupus in maintaining her natural health program.

HOW MUCH SALT DO YOU NEED?

We all know that too much salt in the diet contributes to the development of hardened arteries, high blood pressure, and other ailments. It's the *sodium* in salt that does the damage. Sodium is an essential nutrient, however, and your body needs a certain amount for good health. If you are a normal, healthy person, you can get all the sodium you need from fresh, natural foods. Even if you do not use any salt at all, a good diet will supply from 2,000 to 3,000 milligrams of sodium a day—enough to balance the potassium in your diet. You do not need any additional sodium unless you are perspiring heavily in work or in athletic activities.

Persons suffering from hypertension, water retention, and certain other diseases might be put on a low-sodium diet that restricts the use of sodium-rich foods as well as the use of table salt. Most low-sodium diets supply around 1,000 milligrams of sodium. Such diets should not be used except under the supervision of a physician. You can, however, eliminate table salt and salted foods on your own if you have high blood pressure or water-logged ankles. Lois K. had a blood pressure of 190 over 100, and her ankles were constantly swollen with water (edema). "When I eliminated salt from my diet," she said after attending one of our lectures, "my blood pressure dropped to normal and the swelling in my ankles disappeared. Best of all, I was able to quit taking blood pressure medicine!"

You can check for edema by pressing your thumb against your ankle. If a dent remains in the flesh after you remove your thumb, you have edema. There are many causes of edema, however, so be sure to check with your doctor.

It's important to remember that any additive or preservative such as sodium benzoate, sodium proprionate, monosodium glutamate, or sodium nitrate, that contains sodium is as harmful as salt. If you're cutting down on salt, you should also avoid refined and processed foods that contain sodium additives.

How to Cut Down on
Your Total Sodium Intake

The average American is consuming from 6,000 to 18,000 milligrams of table salt or sodium chloride each day. Since table salt is about 40 percent sodium, this means that salt alone is supplying from 2,400 to 7,200 milligrams of sodium—in addition to the sodium supplied by natural foods and by sodium additives. In some parts of the country, the *drinking water* has a high sodium content, especially where it has been treated with water softeners. The sodium content of processed and preserved foods is so high that no one knows for sure how much sodium an individual may be getting from such foods. It has been estimated that about *65 percent* of the sodium consumed by the average American comes from processed convenience foods. This is undoubtedly one reason why so many Americans are suffering from water retention and high blood pressure.

When the U.S. Senate published the 1st Edition of *Dietary Goals for the United States* (February, 1977), it recommended that salt

TV's "Space Academy" star *Jonathan Harris* has learned to use combinations of vegetables and cooking methods that provide tasty dishes with minimum use of table salt. Properly cooked, most vegetables have a naturally sweet or salty taste.

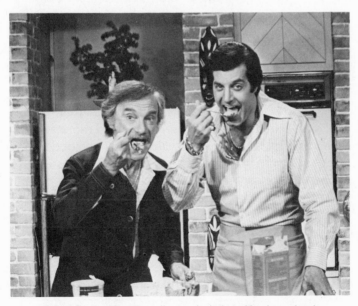

TV's "Space Academy" star Jonathan Harris maintains that meals are tastier as well as more healthful when they are prepared with natural foods.

consumption be reduced to about three grams a day (3,000 milligrams), which would supply about 1,200 milligrams of sodium. Three grams of salt is about three-fifths of a teaspoon. The 2nd Edition of *Dietary Goals for the United States* (December, 1977) recommended that salt intake be reduced to about *five grams* a day. Actually, you can get all the sodium you need from fresh, natural foods. You don't need the sodium supplied by table salt. If you do use table salt, you should be especially careful not to eat processed foods that contain salt or sodium additives. Pretzels, potato chips, salted nuts, and other salted snacks should be avoided whenever possible. Meats, fish, processed cheese, pickles, and other foods that have been pre-seasoned or treated with salt should also be avoided.

Even if your blood pressure is normal and you aren't overweight, an excessive amount of sodium in your diet can lead to heart trouble and other problems by upsetting the balance of sodium and potassium in your blood. Processing a food usually decreases its potassium and increases its sodium. If you eat processed foods instead of fresh, properly prepared foods, you cannot possibly maintain the proper ratio of sodium to potassium in your body.

ADDITIVES AND HEADACHES

If you hear some of your friends say that eating a hot dog gives them a headache, don't laugh. Some people *do* develop headaches after eating foods containing salt or sodium additives—and it could happen to you. Sodium nitrate preservatives and monosodium glutamate seasoning, for example, like salt or sodium chloride, can trigger a migraine headache in susceptible persons. If you are a migraine victim, a handful of salted nuts or potato chips eaten on an empty stomach may cause a headache six to 12 hours later. So if you have been plagued with headaches, try cutting down on the salt, sodium, and nitrites in your diet—or better yet, cut them out completely. The wiener in a hot dog, the great American convenience food, is loaded with sodium nitrite. So are other processed lunch meats. Start reading the labels on the foods you buy if you want to avoid harmful additives.

Malcolm D., a construction worker, suffered from recurring headaches and an occasional irregular heart beat for years before he discovered that the lunch meats he made sandwiches with were the cause of his problems. "I've spent thousands of dollars on doctors trying to find out what was wrong with me," Malcolm complained, "and all the time my trouble was caused by the additives in my food. From now on, I'll put *fresh* food in my lunch pail."

Many serious problems have simple solutions. If you read this book carefully and follow our instructions, you may be able to save yourself a lot of money in medical bills—you'll certainly improve your health.

NITROSAMINES CAUSE CANCER!

Aside from their sodium content, sodium nitrites and nitrates can have potentially lethal effects on your body. Both nitrates and nitrites, for example, undergo chemical changes in your stomach to form nitrosamines, which are known to cause cancer. Frying meats containing nitrites also forms cancer-causing chemicals. Bacon and sausage, American's favorite breakfast meats, are often preserved with nitrites. The next time you experience a rapid heart beat accompanied by headache and flushing of your face, make a list of everything you've eaten over the past 24 hours and see if you've consumed anything containing nitrites or monosodium glutamate.

When you do eat sausage, bacon, wieners, lunch meats, and other foods containing nitrites or nitrates, take a Vitamin C tablet with your meals. Vitamin C blocks the formation of nitrosamines in your stomach. About 500 milligrams of Vitamin C would be more than adequate.

MORE ABOUT SUGAR, FAT, AND REFINED CARBOHYDRATES

You already know from reading Chapter 1 that too much sugar, fat, and refined carbohydrates in your diet can cause disease as well as build up excess body fat. The average person consumes equal amounts of fat and sugar each year along with great quantities of refined carbohydrates. Even if you aren't overweight, *you should cut your fat to a minimum and avoid sugar and refined carbohydrates as much as possible in order to protect your arteries.*

Most people today are getting about 60 percent of their calories from fat, sugar, and refined carbohydrates. Actually, you should be getting 60 percent of your calories from fresh fruits, vegetables, and whole-grain products, which are *natural carbohydrates.* Only about 25 percent of your total calories should be coming from fat, with equal amounts of fat coming from animal sources and vegetable sources. Cutting down on animal fat will greatly reduce your intake of cholesterol. And you'll need only a small amount of vegetable oil to balance the hard fat supplied by meats and other animal products.

Even lean beef and pork are rich in saturated fat, so you should cut consumption of these meats to a minimum and eat more fish and poultry. There is very little fat in fish, and the fat in poultry is mostly in the skin, which can be peeled away. Besides, the small amount of fat found in fish and poultry is largely unsaturated.

In order to make sure that you get all the unsaturated fat you need to balance the animal fat in your diet, use a little cold-pressed vegetable oil (such as safflower oil or corn oil) on a green salad or in a health drink—or you may simply add the oil to foods. A couple of tablespoons a day should be enough. Remember that heating vegetable oil reduces its value as a source of unsaturated fat. So don't depend upon cooked foods for your essential fatty acids.

DIETARY GUIDELINES IN A NUTSHELL

In outlining dietary goals for the United States, the U.S. Senate committee on nutrition recommended these general guidelines for Americans to follow:

1. Increase consumption of fruits and vegetables and whole grains.
2. Decrease consumption of refined and other processed sugars and foods high in such sugars.
3. Decrease consumption of foods high in total fat, and partially replace saturated fats, whether obtained from animal or vegetable sources, with poly-unsaturated fats.
4. Decrease consumption of animal fat, and choose meats, poultry and fish which will reduce saturated fat intake.
5. Except for young children, substitute low-fat and non-fat milk for whole milk, and low-fat dairy products for high-fat dairy products.

6. Decrease consumption of butterfat, eggs and other high cholesterol sources. Some consideration should be given to easing the cholesterol goal for pre-menopausal women, young children and the elderly in order to obtain the nutritional benefits of eggs in the diet.

7. Decrease consumption of salt and foods high in salt content.

You'll learn more in Chapter 10 about how to prepare foods in a healthful way. In the meantime, you can cut down on your consumption of sugar, fat, and refined carbohydrates by making a few simple changes in your everyday eating habits.

TV actor *Tom Hallick* stars in daytime TV's "The Young and the Restless." Ask Tom about the secret of his youthful appearance and he'll tell you that his eating habits have as much to do with his physical appearance as regular exercise.

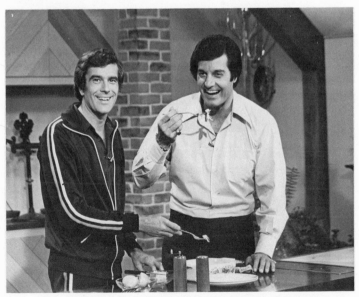

Tom Hallick of daytime television's "The Young and the Restless" controls his body weight by avoiding consumption of refined carbohydrates.

DON'T EAT PROCESSED FOODS

Since processed foods are mostly refined carbohydrates, which are usually loaded with sugar, salt, or saturated fat, you should avoid them as much as possible. Unfortunately, this isn't always easy to do. Since processed foods do not spoil easily and are usually preserved with additives, their long shelf life makes them profitable to sell. So

Some of the lunches offered by fast-food chains are fairly nutritious, but they should not be consumed on a regular basis. The cheese in pizza, for example, is a good food but it is high in fat. And the crust, unless it is made from a whole-grain flour, is high in calories and low in fiber. If you make your own pizza, you can use the flour of your choice. Actress *Barbara Feldon* prefers artichoke flour. "The best pasta is made from artichoke flour," she insists, "which contains lots of protein and little starch."

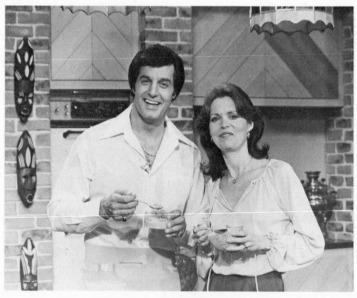

Actress Barbara Feldon prefers balanced meals made up entirely of fresh, natural foods.

they are readily available in convenience food stores. Food advertising is limited almost entirely to promotion of processed foods. You never see television or newspaper advertising promoting the use of fresh fruits and vegetables.

Gloria Swanson makes her own flour by grinding wheat berries. "Around here, we don't have any such thing as flour," she said, affirming her preference for natural foods. "If we want to make anything with wheat flour, we grind our own little berries."

Hamburger patties prepared by fast-food chains often contain "secret" ingredients that alter the taste and texture of the meat—and these ingredients are often artificial additives. Catsup, relish, and other embellishments usually contain sugar. Gooey white-flour buns are composed entirely of refined carbohydrate and artificial additives.

Frying foods greatly contributes to their fat content. Potato chips, for example, are 40 percent fat compared to .1 percent fat in a baked potato. You shouldn't eat fried foods very often. When you do, you should fry the foods yourself in fresh oil and then drain excess oil by placing the still-hot food on absorbent paper. Many fast-food restaurants use the same cooking fat over and over, breaking down the fat until it becomes a gastrointestinal irritant. Very often, the food is literally soaked with grease.

Obviously, you should prepare your foods at home if you want to be sure that everything you eat is wholesome and healthful. It might be all right to eat a hamburger or convenience food occasionally, but it would be better to carry your own lunch whenever you aren't able to eat at home.

HOW THE STARS EAT AWAY FROM HOME

Many of our health-conscious celebrity friends carry their own lunches when they travel or eat away from home. Broadway star *Carol Channing*, for example, carries a lunch of fresh, natural foods with her wherever she goes. She does so to avoid possible allergic reactions to additives in foods. "Since developing an allergy to hair bleach years ago," she explained, "I haven't been able to tolerate any chemicals. So, wherever I go, I carry along a Hammacher Schlemmer thermos and a Mark Cross bag. In the thermos there's pure water, and the bag contains the food I'll have at that particular meal."

Dr. Joyce Brothers takes along yogurt and fresh fruit when she travels.

America's newest singing star, *Debby Boone,* also finds it difficult to eat properly while traveling. And after winning an Oscar for the "Best Song of the Year," she is spending more and more of her time on the road. Once a coffee and sugar addict, she now prefers "real food," which she describes as *natural* and often *raw* foods. "It's really hard to find raw products when you're traveling," she complains. "So I have a tendency not to eat much when I'm on the road."

Debby sticks primarily to salads and baked or broiled chicken when she's traveling. And to further cut down on her intake of fat, she always peels the skin off the chicken.

"God, I believe, wants us to take good care of our bodies," Debby says with conviction. "Our health is important to the Creator. It's great to pray, 'Help me to feel better,' but if you're eating a lot of garbage, especially if you know better, then you're just kidding yourself. A lot of people don't know about nutrition, don't know that it's the best way."

JOIN THE TREND BACK TO NATURAL FOODS

More and more people are becoming aware of the importance of eating properly, and the trend toward the use of natural foods is rapidly gaining momentum. Health food restaurants are popping up everywhere, and grocery stores are carrying more food items that do not contain additives or preservatives. Many packaged foods now state on their labels: "Completely natural. No artificial anything!"

When you cannot find a good restaurant where you can get a good, nutritious meal that is low in fat and sugar, try the nearest grocery store. All super markets now stock yogurt, whole-grain bread, cottage cheese, fresh fruits, raw vegetables, skimmed milk, juices, nuts, and other basic natural foods that can be eaten without cooking. When you're traveling by car, you would be better off eating from a grocery store than in the average restaurant. You won't fall dead if you snack on junk food occasionally, but persons following the *Peter Lupus Body-Improvement Program* are advised to eat properly *consistently* whenever possible.

Turn back to Chapter 1 and review the material on how to balance the foods in your diet. Then make a special effort to eat properly at work and away from home as well as at home, with emphasis on fresh, natural foods at every meal.

A good diet is an important part of the beauty program of supermodel *Cheryl Tiegs.* "I try to stick to natural foods as much as I can," she said in describing her health-and-beauty program. "I never have any canned vegetables. I *always* eat everything fresh."

AVOID HYDROGENATED VEGETABLE OIL

In your effort to cut down on saturated animal fat, remember that vegetable oil that has been hardened or hydrogenated to form

Hydrogenated peanut butter and other processed foods will not spoil readily. But if you keep a supply of fresh, natural foods refrigerated as comedienne *Alice Ghostley* does, you can prepare take-out lunches that are as healthful as meals eaten at home.

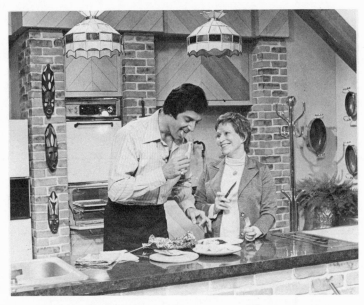

Alice Ghostley, co-star of the movie "Grease," takes her favorite health food dishes with her wherever she goes.

margarine is also a saturated fat. So go easy on the use of margarines. Most commercially prepared snack foods, baked goods, and synthetic toppings are made with hydrogenated vegetable oil, shortening, or some other form of hard fat. (The flakier the crust the harder the fat.) Non-dairy creamers are usually made from coconut oil or palm oil, which are saturated fats mixed with additives.

If you must occasionally use cream in your coffee, whipped cream on your strawberries, or butter on your toast, use the real thing. The synthetic products are less nourishing and just as saturated as the natural products. Furthermore, the additives in a synthetic product may be more dangerous to your health than the saturated fat or cholesterol supplied by butter or cream. The important thing is to cut down on the use of all kinds of fats.

When you buy peanut butter, get the natural variety offered in health food stores. The peanut butter found in most grocery stores has been hydrogenated so that the peanut oil won't rise to the top of the jar. This converts the soft, healthful peanut oil to a hard, harmful fat that is similar to animal fat.

CIGARETTES, COFFEE, ALCOHOL, AND SOFT DRINKS

Many people who try to eat properly unwittingly sabotage their good intentions with daily use of cigarettes, coffee, alcohol, and soft drinks. There is a great deal to be said for moderation in any health habit, good or bad. But if you want the best for your body, you should draw the line on certain bad habits, such as cigarette smoking, and abstain *completely.*

STAY AWAY FROM CIGARETTE SMOKE!

We all know that nothing good can be said about cigarettes. There are 15 or more cancer-causing chemicals in cigarette smoke that can cause cancer in the mouth, throat, liver, intestines, kidneys, and bladder as well as in the lungs. The nicotine absorbed from cigarette smoke stimulates the heart, constricts the blood vessels, and raises blood pressure, contributing to death caused by heart and vascular disease. According to the National Cancer Institute, about 90 percent of all lung cancer is related to cigarette smoking. So is 80 percent of all emphysema and 30 percent of all coronary heart disease. And that's not all. Every cigarette you smoke destroys about 25 milligrams of Vitamin C in your blood. There is now some evidence to indicate that lack of adequate Vitamin C contributes to clogging of arteries. Cigarette smokers are twice as likely to die before middle age as nonsmokers.

Every year, about 300,000 Americans die from diseases related to cigarette smoking. In addition to contributing to the development of such diseases as cancer, stomach ulcers, emphysema, bronchitis, and stroke, cigarette smoking speeds the aging process by decreasing the supply of oxygen to the tissues of your body. With nicotine constricting blood vessels and carbon monoxide displacing oxygen in your blood cells, your body is in double jeopardy.*

Smoking Is a Drug Addiction!

An entire book could be written on the effects of cigarette smoking on the body—a real horror story. We do have some good news for smokers, however. If you smoke and you don't already have cancer or some other disease caused by smoking, you can regain your health if you quit smoking *now.* It may take up to 10 years for an ex-smoker to regain the life expectancy of a non-smoker, but beneficial effects can be seen within a few weeks after smoking is discontinued.

Unfortunately, many people become so addicted to nicotine that they find it difficult to quit smoking. When you consider the damage that smoking does to your body, the decision to quit smoking should not be difficult to make. Once you make that decision, all you have to do is *quit!*

When *John Wayne* lost a lung to cancer after smoking six packs of cigarettes a day for many years, he quit smoking. "I licked the big

---

*The January, 1979, Surgeon General's report on smoking states that "cigarette smoking is far more dangerous to health than we believed in 1964" (when the first Surgeon General's report was released).

C," he told the world. "I caught it early. I was lucky. I hope my story will get other people out for checkups with their docs so that some poor soul can be as lucky as I was." John Wayne's cigarette-related cancer did not recur, but he died of stomach cancer on June 11, 1979, fifteen years after his bout with lung cancer.

You may not be as lucky as John Wayne was in surviving lung cancer or some other cigarette-related disease. So don't wait until you are at death's door to quit smoking. *Quit now!* Don't jeopardize your body program—and your health—by inhaling cigarette smoke. Stay out of smoke-filled rooms. Inhaling smoke from someone else's cigarette may be as bad as smoking the cigarette yourself.

Ted Knight has a legitimate complaint about public smokers. "When I go into a restaurant and see all the people puffing away," he says, "it just infuriates me. Such smokers are not considerate of other people, some of whom may have emphysema, asthma, or a delicate respiratory system. I personally don't want to breathe someone else's cigarette smoke. Slip-stream smoking may be *worse* than actually smoking the cigarette, because the paper is burning." If you smoke, try to follow Ted Knight's suggestion and at least avoid exposing other people to the smoke from your cigarettes.

BE CAUTIOUS WITH ALCOHOL

Alcohol supplies calories and has medicinal value as a nervous system depressant (just the opposite of cigarettes, which act as a stimulant), but it also destroys B vitamins in your body. Many people use alcohol as a social lubricant and to ease nervous tension. Some genuinely enjoy the taste of alcoholic beverages. Regular or daily use of alcohol, however, can develop into an addiction to alcohol, which can lead to disability or death.

Doctors occasionally prescribe alcohol to "improve circulation" by dilating blood vessels. Blood studies, however, indicate that drinking alcohol increases the amount of fat in the blood, particularly triglycerides and low-density lipoprotein. You know from reading Chapter 2 that triglycerides and low-density lipoprotein both contribute to hardening and clogging of the arteries.

So while it might be all right to have a drink occasionally, you should never drink on a regular basis. The minute you feel that you *need* a drink, you should vow never to touch the stuff again. Your liver can dispose of the alcohol supplied by an occasional drink but too much alcohol can overload your liver and deplete your body of B vitamins and other nutrients. Heavy drinking also results in loss of magnesium through the kidneys, contributing to the nervous irritability experienced during a hangover. The average 150-pound man can metabolize about two-thirds of an ounce of straight whiskey or eight ounces of beer in an hour.

Unfortunately, most people who drink alcohol drink too much— so much in fact, that it averages out to *2.7 gallons each year for every man, woman, and child in America.*

Alcohol Contributes to Weight Gain

If you are overweight, you should avoid alcohol completely. Alcohol supplies seven calories per gram, second only into fat in its number of calories. (Fat supplies nine calories per gram. Protein and carbohydrate each supply four calories per gram.) When you drink alcohol, your body burns the alcohol for energy and *stores* the calories supplied by food. When your energy needs are met by alcohol, you are less likely to eat adequate amounts of nutritious foods. Furthermore, your *body* must supply the B vitamins and other nutrients needed to metabolize alcohol.

Adding alcohol to your meals contributes to weight gain by adding calories. Alcoholics who get all their energy from alcohol and do not eat food may not gain weight but their health deteriorates rapidly.

A five-ounce glass of wine supplies about 100 calories. A martini supplies a whopping 220 calories, and a 12-ounce can of beer about 170 calories. "Moderate" drinkers often consume enough alcohol to supply about 1,000 calories a day, making it impossible to lose weight without depriving the body of nutritious food.

How to Stay Out of the Army of Alcoholics

There are more than 10 million alcoholics in the United States. If you are one of these, you can kick the habit if your really want to. Doctors will tell you that if you have a good enough reason to stop drinking, you *can* stop drinking. We cannot think of a better reason to give up alcohol than to cultivate good health and an attractive body that will reward you with a long, active, and happy life. Waiting until you are at death's door for sufficient reason to quit drinking does not make any sense at all. If you have a family, you owe it to *them* to abstain from alcohol. It's simply a matter of caring for yourself and for others. *No matter how long you've been drinking, you can quit if you really want to.* After 10 years of addiction to alcohol, television actor *Gavin MacLeod* quit drinking in order to preserve his marriage. (See Chapter 11 for an in-depth interview with the *new* Gavin MacLeod.)

Actor *Jason Robards* quit drinking after *50 years* of regular use of alcohol. "These days, I have a lot more peace for myself," he notes with a sense of relief. "I choose to care about people. I also choose not to drink . . . . It feels good. It feels as I've gone back to all the things about home and family that were good about my past." Now starring in a remake of the movie "Hurricane," Jason Robards continues to be one of the nation's finest actors.

If you attend a great many social functions, you may have to *bluff* your way through the cocktail hour to avoid pressure from your drinking friends. "Body Shop" guest *Dr. Joyce Brothers* has found a simple way to avoid drinking alcohol at parties. "When I go to cocktail parties," she explained, "I sip a glass of club soda with a twist of lemon in it. It gives me something to do with my hands. Others think I'm having some gin or vodka mixture—and it never goes to my head."

"Tonight Show" host *Johnny Carson* who drank only occasionally at social functions, quit drinking completely when he found that a couple of drinks had adverse effects on his behavior. "I gave up drinking a couple of years ago," he said. "I couldn't handle it." Many people could avoid potential alcoholism if they had the courage to admit that they cannot handle alcohol.

GO EASY ON COFFEE AND COLAS

Coffee and colas are the two most popular beverages in America. One of the reasons for their popularity may be that both contain caffeine, a nervous system stimulant that provides an immediate lift. But caffeine is a drug, and it can be addictive. There are many regular coffee and cola users who feel that they cannot function without their daily dose of caffeine. Some actually suffer from headache and other withdrawal symptoms when they don't have their morning cup of coffee. Since caffeine is a vasoconstrictor, that is, it constricts or narrows blood vessels, the blood vessels around the brain *dilate* when they do not receive their usual caffeine stimulation. This results in the throbbing vascular headache that can be relieved immediately with coffee or caffeine tablets.

In addition to the stimulating effect that caffeine has on the nervous system, it also provides energy by stimulating the adrenal glands, which trigger the release of fatty acids and glucose into the blood stream. If you happen to suffer from hypoglycemia because of an overly sensitive pancreas, however, the sudden rise in blood sugar will be followed by a drastic *fall* in blood sugar a few hours later. This will result in the weakness, nervousness, and hunger that sends you rushing back to the coffee pot time after time. A craving for sweets caused by a fall in blood sugar leads to snacking, overweight, and sugar addiction in a vicious cycle that could destroy your health.

Disease and Coffee Addiction

There is now some evidence to indicate that caffeine may contribute to the development of stomach ulcers, bladder cancer, heart disease, and nervous system disorders. It's well known that caffeine constricts blood vessels and speeds the heart rate. These effects can be deadly in persons suffering from heart disease. The stimulation of the caffeine can turn a mild heart attack into a fatal spasm by decreasing the flow of blood to the heart muscle. Obviously, persons with heart trouble should not drink coffee.

If you are healthy, it might be all right to have a cup of coffee occasionally in order to "perk you up." Do your body a favor, however, and don't drink coffee regularly. One cup of brewed coffee contains from 100 to 125 milligrams of caffeine. Many people drink several cups of coffee every day, which adds up to a dangerous dose of caffeine.

Drink vegetable juices, unsweetened fruit juices, and other healthful beverages during "coffee breaks." When you are thirsty, drink *water.*

Colas May Be Worse Than Coffee!

At the present time, people are consuming more cola than coffee. Since colas are always sweetened, they may be just as bad or worse than coffee. The use of sugar in beverages accounts for over one-fifth of the total amount of sugar used in the United States! A 12-ounce can of soft drink contains about 10 teaspoons of sugar. With sugar-rich caffeine-laden soft drinks heading the list of beverages used by Americans, it's no wonder that so many Americans are overweight.

Children are especially susceptible to the effects of caffeine supplied by colas. Many cola-guzzling youngsters suffer from headache, nervousness, and other symptoms caused by caffeinism. One eight-ounce can of cola contains about 30 milligrams of caffeine. A five-ounce cup of cocoa or hot chocolate may contain up to 50 milligrams of caffeine, and a chocolate bar about 25 milligrams of caffeine. (Tea also contains caffeine.)

A child who has coffee or cocoa for breakfast, a cola for lunch, a chocolate bar for dessert, and who drinks cola to relieve his thirst is bound to be nervous or hyperactive. Add all this up—the nervous stimulation and the fluctuating blood sugar—and you have unpredictable children who are difficult to control. They are also on their way to becoming sick, crippled adults.

How Debby Boone
Kicked the Coffee Habit

Singer *Debby Boone* was a coffee addict as a teenager. But she kicked the habit before her 21st birthday. And she hopes her experience will help prevent some other teenager from becoming similarly addicted. "I just could not do without coffee," Debby revealed. "I literally got sick without it . . . . I got to the point where I was taking a huge thermos of it to Bible school."

Debby could not go without coffee longer than two hours without developing a headache. She literally drank coffee all day long. "I sometimes got to the point where I couldn't sign my name on checks because my hand was shaking so much," she admitted.

Facing the realization that her coffee habit was destroying her health, Debby resolved to quit drinking coffee. "It was terrible," she recalled describing her ordeal. "It was like what I'd heard drug withdrawals were like—chills, shakes, real bad pain. I had to lie in bed for three days. My headaches were so intense, I couldn't even lift my head."

Today, Debby Boone is beautiful, healthy, and successful, and she is a dedicated health enthusiast. Consider Debby's experience and don't take the use of coffee lightly, especially in the case of children.

SUMMARY

1. Many of the leading causes of death and disease could be eliminated simply by making a few changes in everyday health habits.

2. Excessive consumption of sugar, salt, fat, additives, and refined carbohydrates has been linked to six of the ten leading causes of death.

3. You should cut consumption of animal fat to a minimum and try to avoid the use of sugar, salt, and refined carbohydrates.

4. Increase your intake of *natural* carbohydrates so that you get 60 percent of your calories from fruits, vegetables, and whole-grain products.

5. Remember that processed convenience foods often contain hidden sugar and fat as well as refined carbohydrate and synthetic additives.

6. Margarine or hydrogenated vegetable oil may be more harmful to your body than a small amount of natural butter or cream.

7. Cigarette smoking is probably the single most dangerous bad habit of them all.

8. Excessive consumption of alcohol can lead to addiction that results in illness ranging from psychosis to cirrhosis of the liver.

9. The caffeine supplied by coffee and colas has harmful stimulating effects on the body.

10. Rest, exercise, emotional tranquility, and other components of a good health program are just as important as a good diet.

5

How to Cultivate Star-Quality Skin and Hair

Your skin and hair have as much to do with your physical appearance as your body shape. They also accurately reflect deficiencies inside your body. In fact, since skin and hair must receive nourishment from inside your body, the quality of both depends primarily upon the state of your health. Without good health, your body cannot possibly grow healthy skin and beautiful hair. All the cosmetics and beauty products in the world cannot hide unhealthy skin and hair.

"I think the condition of one's hair shows the condition of one's general health," says *Princess Grace of Monaco.* "Products can't do much if you're not healthy."

Toni Tennille agrees. "The *real* key to beautiful hair," she emphasizes, "is a healthy, wholesome, natural diet."

Lynda Day George told us that "A good balanced diet—avoiding sugar, additives, and fat—is your best bet for good skin. And keeping your skin *clean* is important!"

We all know that good grooming is important. Failure to clean the skin adequately, for example, could lead to infection, blemishes,

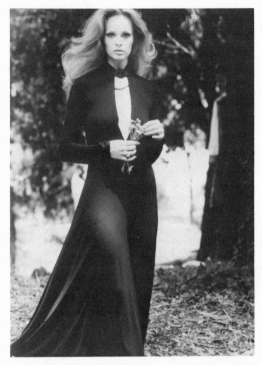

*Actress Lynda Day George, who starred in the TV movie
"Rich Man, Poor Man," occasionally conditions her hair
with mayonnaise in order to restore oil after swimming.*

odor, and other problems. Hair that is not properly cleaned and styled can be a minus instead of a plus to your physical appearance. So while good health may be the first requirement for cultivating attractive skin and hair, good grooming is equally important. Celebrities on the *Peter Lupus Body-Improvement Program* are all aware of the importance of both health and grooming in caring for their skin and hair.

THE SKIN IS AN ORGAN!

If you lose the hair on your head, your physical appearance will suffer but you'll go right on living. Your skin, however, is an important *organ*. It helps protect your body from injury by warning you with pain. It controls your body temperature by responding to the conditions in your environment. The chemical and physical barriers of healthy skin help prevent infection by fighting bacteria. Your skin also eliminates waste. If this function of elimination were hindered by sealing the pores of your skin, your body would die.

Your skin is also a sexual organ. When your mate caresses your body, your skin's erogenous zones provide you with exciting stimulation. If your skin is clean and healthy, the sight and feel of your body will greatly excite your partner.

Obviously, having beautiful and healthy skin and hair, in addition to reflecting your way of life, is an important factor in personal happiness. If you must present yourself before the public, the appearance of your skin and hair may even have a great deal to do with how popular you are.

There are many reasons why you should pay as much attention to your skin and your hair as you do to your body weight and your muscles. If you want to feel good about yourself and look good to others, you *must* cultivate healthy skin and hair and then groom both properly.

BETTER NUTRITION FOR
BETTER SKIN AND HAIR

Since the quality of your skin and hair depends primarily upon receiving nourishment from inside your body, the first thing you should do in cultivating the kind of skin and hair you need for an attractive body is to eat properly. *A deficiency in any nutrient can result in skin and hair problems.* Your skin, hair, and nails are composed primarily of protein, so lack of adequate protein would affect all these structures. There are many specific nutrients needed for healthy skin and hair, but it's *vitamins* that are most often deficient. According to *Human Nutrition,* published by the U.S. Department of Agriculture, "Changes in the skin and hair are often the first indication of nutritional deficiency. ... Vitamins are the nutrients most often implicated in unhealthy appearance of hair and skin."

In the early stages of a nutritional deficiency, hair may lose its glossy appearance and be easily plucked. The skin may become dry, inelastic, and pale in appearance. Probably the most important vitamins for healthy skin and hair are Vitamins A, C, and B complex.

The Case of Julie S.

The experience of Julie S. provides us with a good example of what can happen to skin and hair when there is an advanced nutritional deficiency. Julie was suffering from a chronic eczema-like skin condition that had defied diagnosis and treatment by medical specialists. Also, her hair was falling out and breaking off at the scalp, and it was growing so slowly that breakage alone was thinning her hair. A look at Julie's diet revealed obvious nutritional deficiencies. She was also taking birth control pills and drinking heavily, further draining her body of nutrients.

The solution to Julie's problem was simple. We recommended a balanced diet (see Chapter 1), took her off birth control pills, advised her not to drink (see Chapter 4), and suggested that she supplement her diet with high-potency Vitamin B complex, 1,000 milligrams of Vitamin C, 10,000 units of Vitamin A, and wheat germ oil for essential fatty acids. It took only a few months for Julie's skin to clear up, and it was soon obvious that her hair was growing normally and filling in thickly.

"If I had only known five years ago what I have learned from you," Julie said gratefully, "I could have avoided all the misery and embarrassment of having bad skin. With clear skin and healthy hair, I feel that I have been given a new start in life. Thank you!"

The solution to your skin and hair problems may be simple, too. Every case is different, however, so be sure to read this entire book for guidance in solving your health problems—and check with your doctor. Almost any bad health habit can affect your skin. So it's important to follow a good all-around health program.

Vitamin A and Your Skin

When there is a Vitamin A deficiency, the skin becomes dry, rough, and goose-bumpy. The recommended daily allowance for Vitamin A is about 5,000 units. Some doctors believe, however, that many of us need four times that much for good health. Blood studies indicate that many people are taking in *less* than 5,000 units daily. Large doses of Vitamin A can be toxic, but anyone can safely take up to 25,000 units in a daily supplement for several months.

If you are having skin problems, it might be a good idea to try taking a little Vitamin A to see if you can detect any improvement. Since Vitamin A is a fat-soluble vitamin, persons on a low-fat diet often do not get enough Vitamin A—and just about everyone these days is on a diet.

Note: Since Vitamin E protects Vitamin A in your body, you should probably also take a few hundred units of Vitamin E along with Vitamin A. Wheat germ oil is a rich natural source of Vitamin E as well as the essential fatty acids you need for healthy skin.

You Need All the B Vitamins for Healthy Skin

Riboflavin, niacin, pyridoxine (B_6), and pantothenic acid are believed to be the most important B vitamins as far as the skin is concerned. It's well known that a deficiency in riboflavin, niacin, or pyridoxine can cause such skin diseases as pellagra and seborrhea. Deficiencies in riboflavin, inositol, and other B vitamins may also contribute to loss of hair. A deficiency in practically any B vitamin can have some effect on the skin. And since all the B vitamins work together, *it's always best to take Vitamin B complex rather than a single B vitamin.* Besides, taking only one B vitamin can result in a deficiency in other B vitamins.

Try taking up to 50 milligrams of each of the B vitamins (*micrograms* in the case of B_{12}, biotin, and folic acid) in a B complex formula. Your kidneys will eliminate the B vitamins your body does not use (possibly turning your urine bright yellow).

Brewer's yeast is a good natural source of B vitamins. *Candice Bergen* takes yeast tablets for her skin. "I've been taking yeast pills for years," she said recently in revealing the secret of her beautiful hair. *Liza Minnelli* takes Vitamin B shots. "A Vitamin B_{12} shot every night when I'm working really helps my hair look healthy," she claims.

Vitamin C Holds Your Skin Together

Vitamin C is essential for good skin, since it strengthens the collagen that holds tissue cells together. It also strengthens the tiny blood vessels that supply the skin with nutrients. When there is a deficiency in Vitamin C, the skin bruises easily and injuries heal slowly. Anyone can benefit from taking 500 milligrams of Vitamin C daily. If you suffer from gouty arthritis or kidney stones of the oxalate variety, you may have to be cautious about taking larger amounts of Vitamin C.

You know from reading Chapter 4 that alcohol destroys B vitamins, while smoking destroys Vitamin C. If you drink and smoke, you should take vitamin supplements to protect your skin. Many people who smoke develop "crow's feet" or lines at the corners of their eyes, which are believed to be the result of collagen damage from the effects of nicotine.

Swallowing drugs and medicines can create a vitamin or mineral deficiency in spite of a good diet. Various cold remedies, for example, may deplete Vitamin A reserves. Aspirin forces the body to excrete Vitamin C. Cortisone drugs destroy the zinc you need for a good complexion and for the healing of injuries. Birth control pills zap important B vitamins as well as Vitamin C and zinc, and so on. Try to avoid using drugs and medicines except when absolutely necessary. You'll have a better chance of having good skin if you keep your body clean and your system pure.

A Balanced Diet Is Important

Even if you take supplements, you should not attempt to replace foods with supplements. It's very important to eat a balanced diet of natural foods to get all the nutrients you need for healthy skin and hair. Vitamin supplements will not prevent the premature aging and loss of hair that occurs when a diet is deficient in protein and calories. And without the iron and other minerals you need for healthy blood cells, your skin won't have a healthy glow. So eat properly and *then* supplement your diet to meet special needs. Remember that drinking alcohol and other unhealthy beverages may drain nutrients from your body. *Suzanne Somers* observed that when she quit drinking coffee, tea, and alcohol her complexion improved! Don't sacrifice nutrients by drinking non-nutritious beverages, even if you eat well.

MOISTURIZE YOUR SKIN FROM INSIDE

Drying of the skin from sunbathing and swimming is such a problem that most beach bathers pack moisturizing creams along with suntan lotions. What most of us fail to realize, however, is that pool water or ocean water, like sunlight, *dehydrates* your body by drawing water from your skin. The only way to replace this water is to *drink* water. When you spend the day swimming or sunbathing, drink plenty of water. Finish the day with a cool tub bath and then rub your skin with oil to relieve surface dryness and to prevent further evaporation of moisture from your skin.

Cheryl Tiegs, the highest paid model in the world, drinks large amounts of water to keep her skin plump, moist and free of wrinkles. "I use water to moisturize my skin from the inside out," she said in describing her beauty program. "I drink about four huge glasses of water a day, including one big bottle of Evian spring water." Cheryl also drinks plenty of juices, which she extracts from fresh fruits with a juicer.

THE GOOD AND BAD OF SUNBATHING

When most of us think of beautiful skin, we think about a velvety, tanned skin that is free of blemishes and wrinkles. A white person's skin is more attractive when it is lightly tanned, but nothing is more damaging to white skin than excessive exposure to the sun's rays. The pigment in the skin of black people protects them from sunburn to a great extent, and this protection prevents the premature aging and wrinkling caused by the rays of the sun. The skin of a white person, however, has so little protective pigment that the penetrating ultraviolet rays from the sun easily damage the elastic and collagen fibers deep beneath the surface of the skin. This damage causes shrinking and stiffness that result in permanent wrinkles on the surface of the skin. Take a look at the back of a white farmer's neck and you'll see what we mean. The skin on the face, neck and hands of an old person is usually hard and wrinkled, while the skin on the rest of the body remains soft and smooth.

"If you don't believe that sun ages the skin," says actress *Michele Lee,* "pull down your pants and look at your tush. There won't be a wrinkle on it because that's the only part of your body that's not exposed to the sun."

This doesn't mean, however, that you should stay out of the sun completely. An occasional sunbath—just enough to maintain a *light* tan—makes the skin more attractive to look at and touch. Too much sun can be worse than none. A sunburn greatly damages the skin. The trick is to tan your skin with brief, graduated exposures to the sun's rays so that you don't blister. This will give your skin time to accumulate the pigment it needs to protect itself. The ultraviolet rays then will not penetrate deeply enough to do any extensive damage to the collagen beneath the surface of your skin.

When your skin is lightly tanned and has an attractive color, don't stay in the sun any longer than necessary to maintain that tan. Baking yourself with long exposures to the sun in order to acquire and maintain a dark tan is very damaging to your skin. And when the aging process begins to catch up with you, you'll look 20 years older than you really are.

Remember that any part of your body that is constantly exposed to the sun's rays will age rapidly. If you work or play outdoors, protect your face and neck from the sun as much as possible. Follow *Charo's* example and always wear a hat when you're out in the sun.

How to Tan Your Body Safely

If you are a healthy, active person, chances are you'll want to take advantage of the summer months to spend a little time out of doors swimming, fishing, or working in the yard. But to really enjoy the out of doors, you'll have to first condition your skin with graduated exposures to the sun's rays. Otherwise, sunburn, or the threat of sunburn, will make you a summer cripple. So the best thing to do in preparing for outdoor summer activities is to begin exposing your skin to the sun long before your vacation begins or before you shed your clothes on the beach. This way, you can make your body more attractive to the eye as well as protect it from a painful or aging burn.

The first time you expose your entire body to the sun's rays, limit the exposure to about 15 minutes on each side—front and back. You can increase the exposure time by about one-third (or five minutes) each day. After about four days, pigment will begin to darken your skin to protect you from sunburn. You should have a fairly good tan in about a week.

Don't try to rush your tan! The redness produced during the first few days of sunbathing is caused by burning and not by tanning. It takes time for your body to deposit pigment in your skin. Trying to speed your tan by burning your skin will only damage it. If you suffer a sunburn, you won't have any better tan at the end of a week than a person who has used graduated exposures.

Try to stay out of the sun between 11 A.M. and 2 P.M. The burning rays of the sun are more intense in the middle of the day. You'll have a better chance of tanning without damaging your skin if you avoid the noonday sun.

Remember than when you go fishing or visit the beach, the ultraviolet rays reflected from the water or from the sand may result in a burn even if you stay in the shade. On hazy or overcast days, ultraviolet rays may penetrate the atmosphere enough to produce a severe burn.

How to Protect Your Skin
with Sunscreening Agents

Once you have acquired a light tan or increased your exposure time to 45 minutes or an hour, you should not sunbathe longer to acquire a darker tan if you want to avoid aging of your skin. Even tanned skin will burn if it is subjected to an unaccustomed exposure. You should never stay in the sun longer than two hours, no matter how well tanned your skin might be.

When you *must* stay in the sun longer than usual, use a good sunscreen to protect your skin. Suntan lotions containing salicylates, benzophenone, or para-amino-benzoic acid (paba) are the most effective. Those containing *para-amino-benzoic acid* (which is a B vitamin) in a solution of alcohol are probably best. Remember, however, that alcohol is drying. If you have dry skin, use a suntan *oil* that contains paba. In either case, whether you use lotion or oil, apply the screen half an hour or so before going out into the sun. This will give the paba time to attach itself to your skin. Reapply the screen every two hours or after swimming or sweating heavily.

Actress *Stefanie Powers* feels that *ingesting* paba with rutin helps to prevent sunburn. "Since I've been taking rutin and paba," she said, "I find that my skin doesn't burn as much, and I don't have the harmful effects of the sun that I used to have. Of course, I use a sunscreen. But since I have been taking rutin and paba I notice that I don't burn. If I do get slightly red, my skin turns brown, which it never did before. Also, I don't seem to have the dryness of the skin that I used to have."

Don't try to depend on plain oil to prevent sunburn. Mineral oil or baby oil, for example, even when mixed with iodine, will *not* aid tanning or prevent a sunburn. Too much heavy oil on the skin may even produce skin irritation by clogging pores and preventing evaporation of perspiration.

Vegetable oils, particularly sesame seed oil or olive oil, have sunscreening qualities. If you need a screening oil and you don't have one containing paba, go to your kitchen and get a little vegetable oil.

Note: If you suffer a sunburn in spite of everything you do to protect your skin, you can relieve the pain by covering your body with a cool, wet sheet or by soaking in a tub or cool water. Oiling the skin lightly will hold in moisture and help relieve the dryness and stiffness of parched skin.

The Case of the Splotchy Tan

Occasionally, someone who has taken every precaution to prevent sunburn and to acquire a nice, even tan will end up with a mysteriously splotchy tan that is marred by a rash or by numerous dark spots. This is often the result of photosensitivity, which means that something applied to the skin has increased the skin's sensitivity to the sun's rays. Perfumes, deodorant soaps, medicated cosmetics, aftershave lotions, detergents, and a variety of other products can result in photosensitive skin. Lemon and lime juices are especially potent photosensitizers. So are lotions containing lemon or lime essence.

The location of splotchy pigmentation or a skin rash may give you some clue as to the offending agent. If the discoloration is around your hands and arms, and you have been squeezing lime wedges at poolside, then your problem might be lime juice. If a rash develops around your neck, the culprit might be aftershave lotion or perfume. Ingested drugs and artificial sweeteners can sensitize your entire body.

Always see your doctor when you develop a skin problem of any kind. There are many causes of skin rashes and all of them are difficult to diagnose.

HOW TO CLEAN YOUR SKIN AND HAIR

Someone once said that "Cleanliness is next to Godliness." There's no doubt that cleanliness is an important aspect of body care. No matter how slim and fit you are, you won't be physically appealing if your skin is greasy and speckled with blackheads or if it's flaky and wrinkled. A dirty, smelly body is definitely a turnoff when it comes to close association with people, especially the opposite sex. In fact, the response you get from your lover may be determined largely by the appearance and odor of your skin. So be sure to keep your skin clean. "Body cleaning" is an integral part of the *Peter Lupus Body-Improvement Program.*

Cleaning Methods Depend Upon Skin Type

How you clean your skin should depend upon the type of skin you have. If you have normal skin, bathing twice a day with almost any kind of soap is all right. If you have oily skin or dry skin, however, you'll have to use a cleaning procedure that's entirely different from that used by a person with normal skin. There are some people, for example, who should not use soap and hot water on their skin. Others may have to use plenty of soap and water. What's best for one person may not be best for you. Study this chapter carefully before you decide what approach you should use in cleaning your skin.

Actress *Elizabeth Taylor,* one of America's 10 most beautiful women, cleans her skin with soap and water. Singer *Lena Horne* alternates the use of water and baby oil. ABC's "Good Morning America" television beauty expert *Cheryl Tiegs* cleans her skin with cream. "Cleaning with a mild soap and water may be fine for some women," she reported, "but my skin tends to be too dry to put water on it."

You can see that even the beautiful people use different skin-cleaning methods. *Elizabeth Taylor* maintains that any woman can be beautiful with such simple beauty habits as cleaning the skin with soap and water, eating nutritious foods, and shampooing the hair regularly. "Perfect features and a perfect figure are not necessary," she says. "People care more about inner beauty. Beauty is a glow that comes from happiness."

Try to stay happy, but first be clean and healthy. And be sure to exercise regularly to keep your body strong and well developed.

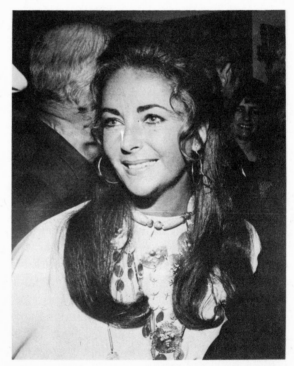

Actress Elizabeth Taylor, one of the world's most beautiful women, practices simple, sensible beauty habits that any woman can follow.

Oily Skin vs. Dry Skin

A dermatologist gifted for simplifying complicated procedures

nce said, "If skin is oily, dry it; if it's dry, oil it." The solution to skin
roblems is not quite as simple as that, but it's pretty close.

It's usually very easy to tell whether you have oily skin or dry skin.
your skin is oily, an excessive amount of skin oil may clog pores to
ause bumps and blackheads. You can test for oiliness by taking a
iece of brown paper bag and rubbing it back and forth across your
orehead several times. If there's enough oil on your skin to make the
aper translucent, your skin may be too oily. Skin that is too dry may
e rough, scaly, and easily irritated. In either case, whether your skin is
ily or dry, improper cleaning methods can lead to serious medical or
osmetic problems.

Cleaning Procedures for Oily Skin

When skin is oily, frequent washing with moderately alkaline soap
such as Ivory) may be necessary to keep the skin pores from
ccumulating oil. And the oilier the skin, the more washing required
nd the more alkaline the soap should be. Persons suffering from
cne caused by excessively oily skin may have to use highly alkaline
cne soaps that have special drying and degreasing qualities. Since
he scalp and the face are the oiliest portions of the body, they may
equire more frequent washing than other portions of the body.

Wash as often as necessary to keep your body clean and your
ores unclogged. Make sure that all of the soap residue is rinsed from
our skin. You may find it necessary to wash your face between baths.
n a pinch, astringents may be used to dissolve accumulating oil.
Rubbing alcohol makes a good astringent. For a little something extra,
ou can mix four ounces of alcohol with four ounces of distilled water
nd one-half teaspoon of alum. Just dab the solution over the oily
ortions of your face, particularly around your nose.

If you want to use a facial mask to dry oily skin, mix two
ablespoons of alcohol with each tablespoon of clay mask to make a
aste. Apply the paste to your face, let it dry, and then wash it off with
varm water. Finish with a cold-water rinse.

Sally Struthers of "All in the Family" makes her own special
stringent by mixing one ounce of apple cider vinegar with eight
ounces of water, which is then refrigerated.

How to Get Rid of Blackheads

Whenever pores accumulate enough oil to form blackheads i spite of regular washing, it may be necessary to employ speci cleaning methods to prevent the development of acne. When o hardens in a pore, oxidation blackens the surface portion of the plug Deterioration of the oil deeper in the clogged pore may produc irritating fatty acids that cause inflammation and swelling. So don ignore pores that are clogged by blackheads.

To clean clogged pores, first wash your skin with soap and wate to remove surface dirt and germs. Apply hot, wet towels to soften th blackheads. Gently press the dark plugs from the pores with you finger tips (don't use your nails!) and then wash again with soap an water to guard against infection. A shower would be best. Dry you face with a *clean* towel. It may be necessary to empty clogged pores a least once a week if your skin is very oily. You should, of course do thi in the evening before retiring so that you won't have to go out in publi with a splotchy face. *Always change pillow cases when you clean you pores.* Otherwise, you may contaminate freshly opened pores.

If you have acne, wash your face and other oily areas frequentl with strongly alkaline soap and hot water—*until your skin is so dry tha it peels.* Rubbing your body with beauty grains or wet corn meal wi remove dead skin and help open clogged pores.

Lynda Day George has a remedy for the occasional skin blemish "I've found that a little lemon juice applied over a 'blossom' will usuall clear the skin," she told us in a personal interview. "If the 'blossom persists, a dab of toothpaste at night seems to do the trick. I don't hav the foggiest idea why this works, but there it is!" (The acidity of lemor juice inhibits bacterial growth. Toothpaste, in addition to sealing ou bacteria, may have antibacterial ingredients.)

When you use cleansing creams to dissolve oil deep in pores always remove the cream by washing with soap and water. Use a much hot water as necessary to remove all traces of cream and oil.

HOW TO CLEAN DRY SKIN

Skin becomes dry when the body does not supply the skin with enough oil to prevent evaporation of moisture through pores. Dry skir does not require as much washing as oily skin. If you have dry skin, you should not wash any more than necessary to remove surface dirt. Too much washing would only remove what little protective oil you have, resulting in increased evaporation of moisture and greater dryness. Excessive use of soap and water, especially hot water, would result in inflammation and cracking of the skin. When you do use soap, it may be necessary to use special low-alkaline, super-fatted soaps that will leave a little oil on the skin.

Persons with severely dry skin may not be able to use any soap at all during the winter when dry, cold outdoor air and dry, heated indoor air increases evaporation of moisture from the skin. It may be necessary to bathe in plain water and then apply moisturizing creams or oils to the skin to hold in the absorbed moisture. If a bath oil is used, the skin should be patted dry so that a thin film of oil remains on the skin.

Doris Day occasionally oils her dry skin with petroleum jelly (Vaseline). Once a week, she covers her body with petrolatum and slips on a flannel nightgown and a pair of socks before going to bed.

Remember that as you grow older your skin tends to become drier. When the years catch up with you, you may have to ease up on the use of soap, even if you've never had a skin problem. Of course, if you have dry skin with small pores, you can clean your skin adequately with cleansing cream at any age.

Note: It's always a good idea to include a little vegetable oil in your diet to make sure that you supply your body with the essential fatty acids it needs to manufacture skin oil. Persons suffering from *true* dry skin, however, which is an inherited disorder, are simply deficient in oil glands. This makes it necessary to apply oil to the *surface* of the skin.

HOW TO HANDLE COMBINATION SKIN

Some people claim to have a "combination skin," which means that some portions of their body may be dry while other portions are oily. It's not unusual, for example, to have a dry face with an oily nose. In this case, it may be necessary to apply a lubricating cream to the face after washing and then dab the nose with alcohol or some other astringent two or three times a day. In portions of the body where the skin is dry and itchy, less soap and water is used. Where the skin is oily, however, soap and hot water may be used freely.

Even if you have normal skin, you might suffer from dryness in the winter and oiliness in the summer. Obviously, it's very important that you learn how to determine for yourself when you should use more or less soap and water as opposed to using oils and moisturizers.

After middle age, the pores around the nose often enlarge with excessive accumulation of oil. If that happens to you, you'll have to pay special attention to your face if you want to prevent the development of huge, unsightly blackheads. Follow the cleaning procedure described earlier for cleaning clogged pores.

HOW TO ELIMINATE BODY ODORS

It's normal to have a certain amount of body odor at the end of the day. *Unpleasant* odors are usually caused by the effect of bacterial activity on perspiration, especially in portions of the body where perspiration does not evaporate freely. Generally, persons with dry skin have less trouble with body odor. If you can keep your skin dry of perspiration, you can usually control body odors. In any event, a daily bath will eliminate unduly offending odors.

The feet, groin, and underarm areas are the most difficult to keep free of bad odors. In addition to being closed off from circulating air, the groin and the armpit secrete perspiration from *apocrine* glands, which cause more odor than the sweat secreted by the eccrine glands in other portions of the body. The apocrine glands are not activated until puberty, and they are less active in old age. This is one reason why children and old people are often able to get by with less bathing.

Even if you have dry skin and you do not often use soap on your body, you may have to use soap at least once daily under your arms and in your groin area as well as on your feet. The eccrine glands are stimulated by heat, but the apocrine glands are activated by emotions as well as by hormones. For this reason, you may have to wash your underarm and groin areas with soap even when you don't exert yourself enough to "work up a sweat."

Be sure to change your clothes daily to prevent accumulation of odor. When necessary, use a good deodorant under your arms. Clipping the hair in your armpits will reduce odor by removing hair that accumulates bacteria and traps waste products.

Note: If commercial underarm deodorants irritate your skin, try using a mixture of corn starch and baking soda.

WHAT ABOUT WRINKLING?

The best way to eliminate wrinkles is to *prevent* them. You already know that overexposure to the sun wrinkles and ages the skin by damaging skin collagen. Nutritional deficiencies, cigarette smoking, and other health-wrecking factors also contribute to the development of wrinkles. Once true wrinkles develop, there's not much that you can do to get rid of them. There are, however, a few things you can do to minimize wrinkles on special occasions.

We have all noticed wrinkling that occurs on our fingertips after spending a long time in water, especially in salt water or chlorinated water. This is dehydration caused by the mineral content of the water. Sun also dehydrates the skin. When the skin over your entire body is dehydrated, old wrinkles are exaggerated and new wrinkles appear. You can remove these wrinkles by drinking plenty of water and by bathing in a tub of cool water containing a few tablespoons of vegetable oil or baby oil. Pat yourself dry after bathing so that a thin film of oil remains on your skin. Or, after a bath, you may rub your skin with oil to hold in absorbed moisture. If it's only your face you're concerned about, you can cover your face with a wet, lukewarm towel for about five minutes and then rub a little oil on your face. Some people use a facial sauna to hydrate the skin of their face—until it is plump with moisture. You can get the same effect by draping a towel over your head to catch the steam from a pot of boiling water.

Almost any kind of oil applied to the skin will prevent evaporation of moisture through pores. Vegetable oil or Crisco may be just as effective as more expensive oils (moisturizers). If you suffer from acne and you do not want to use oil on your skin, you can use a commercial non-oily product to seal in moisture. Any product that contains urea, for example, a chemical that attracts and holds moisture without clogging pores, would work nearly as well as oil.

HOW TO CLEAN YOUR HAIR

How often you wash your hair depends primarily upon how oily your scalp is, how much you perspire, and the amount of dust and dirt you're exposed to. *You should wash your hair as often as necessary to keep it free of dirt, dandruff, or excess oil.* Since the scalp is normally the oiliest portion of the body, it's not likely that you can wash your hair too much. Most people do not wash their hair often enough. Once a week may be often enough for someone who has dry skin, but the average person can benefit from two or more washings a week. If your skin and scalp are oily, you may find it necessary to wash your hair every day. *Liza Minnelli* washes her hair under a shower twice a day.

When expert New York hair stylists *Fred and Vincent Nardi* visited us on the set of "Peter Lupus' Body Shop," they assured us that frequent shampooing will not harm healthy hair. "Wash your hair as soon as it loses its bounce and shine," they advised. "For some people this may be every three days; for others, it may mean every day!"

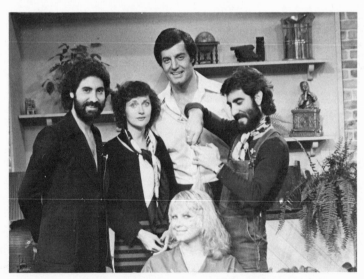

Fred and Vincent Nardi, authors of the book "How to Do Your Own Hair Like a Pro," recommend use of a large, wide-toothed comb when combing wet or tangled hair.

Detergents vs. Soaps

Oily hair should be washed with a detergent shampoo that contains more detergent and less fatty material. *Dry hair* calls for a shampoo that contains more fatty material and less detergent. Since practically all shampoos are detergents, that is, they do not contain soap, you don't have to worry about whether the water you use is hard or soft. Unlike soap, detergents do not combine with the minerals (calcium and magnesium) in hard water to form a dull film on your hair. If a detergent shampoo irritates your skin, however, you should use a soap shampoo. And if the water you use is hard, you may have to use an acid rinse to remove mineral residue from your hair.

To make an acid rinse, squeeze the juice of one lemon into a basin of water or add one tablespoon of white vinegar to each glass of water poured into a basin. After you have rinsed your hair with one of these solutions, a fresh-water rinse will wash away the minerals.

If your hair seems to be dry following a shampoo, you can use a creme rinse or a conditioner to coat your hair with a thin film of oil. Conditioners that contain protein will give thin hair more body by coating it with a layer of protein substance. Always rinse with *cold* water after conditioning fine hair.

Jaclyn Smith of "Charlie's Angels" conditions her hair with mayonnaise. "I put mayonnaise on my hair and then wrap a hot towel around my head," she explained. "After 30 to 40 minutes, I remove the towel and shampoo out the mayonnaise. It makes my hair shiny, gives it luster, and puts back natural oils."

Comb Carefully!

When you are combing your hair following a shampoo, use a wide-toothed comb so that you don't break the wet hair. If you comb your hair while using a hand-held hot-air drier, remember that heated hair breaks easily. Comb gently and carefully. Forceful combing of tangled hair can break hundreds of hairs. Hair that tangles easily should be cut as short as possible to minimize tangling. A conditioner or a creme rinse following a shampoo will help prevent tangling and make combing easier.

If your hair is properly cut and styled to take advantage of its natural growth pattern, it can be groomed with a minimum amount of brushing or combing. *Farrah Fawcett,* star of the movie "Sunburn," is as well known for her beautiful flowing tresses as she is for her gorgeous body. But she doesn't have to spend much time fixing her hair. "The thing that's easiest for me is my hair," she revealed. "It's naturally curly and has lots of body. Even for photography, when makeup can take an hour, my hair takes only ten minutes. I wash it every day, and sometimes I condition it while I'm on the beach."

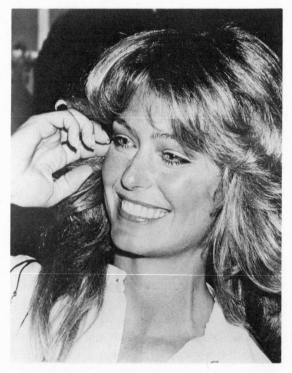

Farrah Fawcett, TV and movie star, is blessed with naturally beautiful hair that requires little care.

You won't have to spend a long time combing or fixing your hair if it is natural and healthy.

HOW TO PREVENT LOSS OF HAIR

Everyone worries about losing hair. In recent years, increasingly large numbers of women have been reporting excessive hair loss. There are probably just as many women who worry about thinning hair as there are men who worry about baldness.

When a man loses hair in the natural pattern of male baldness, there isn't much that can be done about it. But when a man or a woman loses hair over the entire scalp as a result of a nutritional deficiency, improper grooming, and other factors, further loss can be prevented to allow new growth to replace the lost hair.

You learned earlier in this chapter that a deficiency in protein, vitamins, minerals, essential fatty acids, and other nutrients can contribute to loss of hair. When hair has been damaged by harsh alkaline dyes and permanent wave solutions, it may break so easily that light combing results in hair loss. Keep your hair its natural color, and style it so that you don't have to curl or straighten it artificially. *Natural* is best if you want to *keep* your hair.

Make sure that your hair drier does not overheat your hair. Most hair driers, especially those with an Underwriters Laboratory approval label, are equipped with a thermostat to prevent overheating. Keep the drier at least six inches from your hair. *Quit using the drier before your hair is totally dry.*

Charo uses a filter on the blower of her drier so that she can dry her hair with a minimum amount of heat.

Many women—and some men—lose hair as a result of pulling hair too tightly with ponytails, pigtails, or rollers. Constant traction on the hair can break it or cause it to turn loose at the scalp. Generally, hair lost this way will regrow, but repeated or prolonged pulling on the hair may damage hair roots to cause *permanent* hair loss.

Don't Brush Your Hair Away

A certain amount of brushing is good for your hair, but too much can be harmful, especially if you use the wrong kind of brush. A nylon brush with sharp tips, for example, can split or break hair. Hair that has been damaged by bleaching may break like straw when brushed. Assuming that you have strong, healthy hair that can benefit from moderate brushing, brush your hair enough each day to remove skin flakes and other debris and to distribute scalp oil. Use a brush that has *natural* bristles, or at least make sure that the tips of nylon bristles have been rounded. Whatever type of brush you use, don't brush excessively. Forget the 100-strokes-a-day routine. Just enough brushing to keep your hair looking good is enough.

Hair grows about one-half inch a month (six inches a year). Obviously, if you keep breaking hair off at the scalp each day with improper grooming procedures, your hair growth won't replace the lost hair fast enough to prevent thinning. You normally shed about 60 hairs a day. If you see a few hundred hairs on your comb every time you groom your hair, you may be *breaking* your hair.

There are, of course, many causes of hair loss, such as emotional stress, pregnancy, illness, drug therapy, scalp infections, overexposure to X-rays, and so on. Most result in temporary hair loss, but some can lead to permanent baldness. Be sure to see a good dermatologist if you begin to experience sudden or unexplained loss of hair.

SUMMARY

1. Proper care of your skin and your hair will do as much for your physical appearance as exercising your muscles or reducing your body weight.

2. Good nutrition and a clean body are essential in cultivating healthy skin and beautiful hair.

3. A balanced diet of fresh, natural foods, supplemented with Vitamins A, B, and C, will assure an adequate supply of essential nutrients for your skin and hair.

4. The type of cleaning procedure you use on your skin or your hair is determined largely by whether your skin is dry or oily.

5. Oily skin and hair require frequent washing with moderately alkaline soaps and shampoos.

6. Dry skin and hair require less washing, less hot water, and low-alkaline soaps and shampoos that contain a high percentage of fat.

7. Dry skin must be moisturized from the inside and then oiled on the surface to prevent evaporation of moisture through pores.

8. Skin must be tanned in a progressive manner to avoid damaging skin collagen with a sunburn.

9. Facial wrinkles can be temporarily minimized by steaming the face with hot towels and then applying a little oil to hold in absorbed moisture.

10. Forceful combing or brushing of dry or tangled hair, especially while using a hand-held hot-air drier, can damage or break hair.

6

What Celebrities Do to Keep Their Teeth and Nails Strong and Beautiful

Phil R. had beautiful teeth when we first met him at one of our lectures. "Why should I do anything special for my teeth?" he asked in response to our presentation on care of the teeth. "I rarely brush my teeth—and I don't have any cavities. So why should I wear out my teeth brushing them?" When we saw Phil a year later, he had false teeth! That could happen to you, too, if you don't know how to take care of your teeth and your gums. There's more to caring for your teeth than simply *brushing* your teeth. If you want to make sure that you keep *your* teeth, be sure to study this chapter carefully, even if you have "good teeth."

Most books and articles on health have very little to say about teeth. Celebrity interviews almost invariably stress skin, weight, and energy. Yet, the condition of the teeth play an important role in maintaining the health and appearance of the body. And, like the skin, the condition of the teeth may reflect general health as well as personal habits. *Dirty* teeth, for example, in addition to detracting from physical appearance, clearly label a person as either ignorant or careless. Tooth decay casts suspicion upon eating habits. Loss of teeth, for whatever reason, affects health adversely by interfering with ability to chew, making it necessary to eliminate certain healthful foods from the diet. Even if decayed teeth can be capped to improve their appearance or lost teeth replaced by dentures or bridges to aid chewing, there is no satisfactory substitute for natural teeth. So even if you can replace natural teeth with attractive-looking artificial teeth, you cannot afford to ignore your teeth if you want to keep your body strong, healthy, and beautiful. Besides, the misery and expense of extensive dental work should provide enough reason to take good care of your teeth, even if you aren't concerned about your health and your appearance.

TEETH SHOULD LAST FOREVER!

When *Leon Spinks* wrested the world heavyweight boxing crown from *Muhammad Ali,* the new champion's most noticeable physical feature was the absence of his front teeth. Of course, many fighters lose teeth in the ring. And the toothless grin of a football lineman is a mark of the game. But *there is no reason at all why anyone should lose teeth except as a result of injuries or athletics.* The sad truth, however, is that about one-half of all Americans over the age of 55 have no natural teeth. In Great Britain, one of every three persons is toothless by the age of 17!

Many teeth are lost to decay, which erodes the teeth until they collapse or crumble. In America, more teeth are lost to *gum disease* than to all other factors combined. Fortunately, both tooth decay and gum disease can be prevented. A shark grows a new tooth everytime he loses one, and a rabbit's front teeth keep growing, but in your case *a tooth lost is a tooth gone forever.* So take good care of your teeth. They are more valuable to you than all the gold in the world.

HOW TO PREVENT TOOTH DECAY

Although about half of all Americans drink fluoridated water, tooth decay is still rampant. We know that tooth decay is caused by sugar-eating streptococcus bacteria. These germs secrete a corrosive acid that literally dissolves tooth enamel. Only about one American in 100 is immune to tooth decay. If you are one of the lucky ones and your saliva contains the right antibodies, you won't have to worry too much about tooth decay, no matter what you eat. But if bacteria thrive in your mouth, you'll have to make sure that you don't *feed* these bacteria by eating sugar and other refined carbohydrates. And you'll have to keep your teeth clean enough to prevent a build-up of plaque that allows bacteria to attach themselves to your teeth. You may also have to be cautious about kissing persons who have decayed teeth, since such teeth harbor billions of communicable bacteria. It might even be possible to catch or transmit tooth decay! So, for the sake of romance, folks, don't let bacteria invade your teeth. When your teeth and gums are clean and healthy, your mouth is beautiful and exciting. But when your mouth is neglected to the point where your teeth decay and your gums become infected, your mouth becomes a veritable cesspool.

Sugar Is the No. 1 Culprit
in Tooth Decay

In Chapters 1 and 4, you learned that excessive use of sugar contributes to the development of overweight, diabetes, hardened arteries, colon cancer, and other health problems. It has been learned in recent years that the bacteria that erode tooth enamel feed primarily upon *sugar*. It's not so much the *amount* of sugar you ingest as it is the *frequency* of eating sugar. Bathing your teeth with small amounts of sugar-sweetened foods or beverages several times a day, for example, provides frequent feedings for the bacteria lurking in the crevices of your teeth. This is more damaging to your teeth than eating a large amount of sugar once a day. And if the sugar is in the form of syrup, caramel, and other sweets that stick to your teeth, the bacteria can feast continuously. You should try to eliminate refined sweets from your diet. When you do eat sweets, you should brush or rinse your teeth to remove all traces of the sugar. Eating sweets between meals, when you cannot brush your teeth, is never a good idea. Reserve sweets for use as desserts following meals—and then *brush your teeth after each meal.*

Loretta Swit of *M*A*S*H* carries a toothbrush with her everywhere she goes. "I'm religious about dental checkups and brushing my teeth," she said. "I take my toothbrush with me when I'm on location or when I go to the studio. I feel that it's a *necessity* to brush my teeth after each meal. I haven't had a cavity in four or five years."

Sugar Under Any Other Name Is Still Sugar

In 1977, it was estimated that the average American was consuming 129 pounds of sweeteners a year, including syrups, honey, dextrose, and other sweeteners. About 75 percent of all sugar consumption comes from refined or prepared foods, many of which contain *hidden* sugar. So even if you avoid sugar, candy, soft drinks, pastries, and other obviously sugar-sweetened foods, you won't be able to avoid sugar completely unless you eat only fresh, natural foods. Canned peas, for example, might contain sugar.

Read the labels on packaged foods. Under the new labeling law, the list of ingredients on the label of a product names its contents in descending order according to dry weight. The higher on the list the sugar, the greater the sugar content of the product. (Some processed cereals contain more sugar than cereal!) But don't just look for the word "sugar." Look for other names for sweeteners, such as glucose, fructose, invert sugar, corn syrup, and "natural sweeteners." All of these can contribute to tooth decay. Artificial sweeteners may not harm your teeth, but they may be harmful to your body. Try to avoid sweeteners of any kind.

Remember: When you eat anything sweet, processed, or packaged, rinse or brush your teeth to remove food residue. Refined carbohydrates, such as white bread, are also easily fermented by the bacteria in your mouth. So try to avoid white-flour products as well as sugar and other sweeteners.

GUMS REQUIRE SPECIAL CARE

Tooth decay is bad enough, but gum disease is worse. You can at least see decay soon enough to do some patchwork before a large cavity forms. Gum disease, however, creeps up unaware. Very often, the disease is far advanced before it is discovered. It may then be too late to prevent loss of teeth. If you want to *prevent* gum disease, you'll have to clean your teeth and your gums regularly. Even if you're one of those fortunate persons who is not bothered by tooth decay, you'll have to brush your teeth in order to protect your gums. Don't ever skip brushing just because you don't have any cavities.

Not too many years ago, dentists instructed their patients to brush *down* on their top teeth and *up* on their bottom teeth. The idea was to brush food particles away from gum margins and to avoid aggravating receding gums. It turned out, however, that while such brushing cleaned the teeth adequately it did not clean the gum margins enough to prevent gum disease. And here's why: There is normally a shallow groove between the teeth and the gums at the gum margin. If you do not keep this grove clean by brushing under the edges of your gums, plaque, tartar, calculus, and other matter will begin to accumulate under the gum margins. This creeping build-up causes the gum to relax its grip on the teeth, so that deep pockets form between the teeth and the gums. As these pockets grow deeper, bacterial infection begins to erode the tough fibers that anchor the teeth in their bony sockets. Very often, a victim of gum disease may not even be aware of the creeping gum detachment until a tooth becomes so loose that it actually wobbles in its socket. It may then be too late to save the tooth.

Early symptoms of gum disease may be bad breath or a pink toothbrush. The bad breath is caused by decomposition of food particles trapped in gum pockets. A pink toothbrush may point to bleeding from inflamed or infected gums.

The older you become, the more important it is to clean under the edges of your gums. After the age of forty, for example, your gums normally begin to recede or detach from your teeth. If you don't make a special effort to clean the widening crevice at your gum margins, you may not be able to avoid the development of gum disease (pyorrhea or periodontal disease). Once gum disease becomes advanced, gum boils may develop, or pus may ooze from under the gum margins. Bone around the roots of the affected teeth is dissolved. When the teeth become loose, it may be necessary to extract some of them to eliminate deep pockets of infection. Obviously, it's just as important to clean under the edges of your gums as it is to clean your teeth if you want to keep your teeth as long as you live.

Sue D. was 38 years old when she started having trouble with her gums. Recurring gum boils led to extraction of two of her molars (back teeth) before she realized she was in danger of losing her teeth. Her dentist advised her to brush her teeth and use dental floss. We further advised Sue to supplement her diet with Vitamin C and calcium and instructed her in the use of an oral irrigation device. When she returned to her dentist for her six-month checkup, the pockets around her back teeth were clean and free from infection. Her gums were pink and firm instead of red and spongy. "I really believe that the vitamins and irrigations helped," Sue reported. "My dentist says that if my gums stay in such good shape I won't lose any more teeth and I won't have to have gum surgery. The advice you gave me was free, but it was worth a million dollars!"

Surgery, Diets and Vitamins

It's never too late to begin proper teeth-and-gum cleaning procedures. Many people with *advanced* gum disease could save their teeth by brushing properly, irrigating gum pockets, and paying attention to oral hygiene. A periodontist, a dentist who specializes in gum surgery, can cut away gum pockets to make cleaning easier.

See a dentist regularly for a checkup. Have your teeth cleaned once or twice a year by a dental hygienist who can scrape deposits from under the edge of your gums. If you develop problems in spite of regular cleaning, make an appointment with a periodontist for a deep scaling.

Good nutrition is also important. Lack of adequate Vitamin C in the diet will contribute to softening and bleeding of gums. Too much sugar can feed bacterial infections in gum pockets, making it difficult or impossible to control gum disease. *If you have a chronic gum infection, be sure to have your blood sugar checked for diabetes.*

Fad diets that do not supply balanced amounts of essential vitamins and minerals can contribute to the development of gum disease as well as to tooth decay. When there is a calcium deficiency, for example, the bone around the roots of the teeth surrenders calcium for more essential functions, allowing teeth to loosen and pull away from the gums. This will contribute to the development of infection around the roots of the teeth, practically assuring loss of the affected teeth.

An excessive amount of phosphorous in the diet, as in an all-meat diet, drains calcium from your bones, especially your jaw bones. (If you go on a high-protein reducing diet, select a protein powder that you mix with milk—and then eat at least one balanced meal each day.)

Beautiful "soap opera" star *Patty Weaver* supplements her diet with milk-based drinks that keep her teeth and bones strong as well as supply her with the strength and energy she needs for daily television filming.

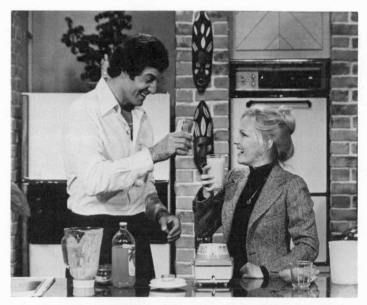

Patty Weaver of television's "Days of Our Lives" and Peter Lupus toast to the healthful benefits of milk as a source of bone-building calcium.

HOW TO BRUSH YOUR TEETH AND GUMS

Most of us grew up believing that a hard brush was best for cleaning the teeth. Today, however, *soft* brushes are recommended. The reason for this switch is that dentists now recognize the importance of brushing under the edges of the gums. You must use a soft brush to do this without injury. To brush properly, angle the brush toward your gum margin so that the bristles of the brush will slip up under the edges of your gums. You may use short back-and-forth strokes or simply move the brush in a tight circular motion. If you prefer, you can use a special gum brush to clean under your gum margins after you have cleansed your teeth with a regular brush.

Selecting a Dentifrice

The more abrasive your dentifrice is the greater its cleaning powers. Soda or salt, for example, make an effective dentifrice. Remember, however, that excessive use of an abrasive dentifrice can wear down the enamel of your teeth. So while it might be all right to use an abrasive powder on your teeth occasionally to remove stubborn deposits, you should use a less-abrasive toothpaste most of the time.

You can find out if you are cleaning your teeth adequately by chewing a tablet of red disclosing dye after brushing your teeth. Plaque or deposits on your teeth will show up as bright red stains. You can purchase red disclosing dye in any drug stores.

Using Toothpicks in a Pinch

You should always try to clean your teeth with a *brush* after eating. When you are unable to brush your teeth, you should at least rinse your teeth with water. Toothpicks or interdental stimulators can be used when a toothbrush is not available. An interdental stimulator is a soft balsawood toothpick that can be pressed between the teeth and against the gum margin. They're great for cleaning teeth and stimulating the gums. Take some along with you when you eat out or go on a trip. You can buy them in any drug store.

If you get caught on a picnic without a toothbrush or a toothpick, you can make one from a tree twig. Just break a match-size twig from a tree (preferably oak) and soften one end by chewing it before using it to clean your teeth—just as grandma used to do.

Regardless of what you do to your teeth during the day, you should never fail to brush your teeth before you go to bed each night. Food particles that remain between the teeth and under gum margins overnight provide bacteria with plenty of fuel for eroding teeth and developing an infection.

USE DENTAL FLOSS ONCE A DAY

No matter how vigorously or carefully you brush your teeth, you won't be able to brush away deposits and food particles wedged between your teeth. You can remove these particles with dental floss, which should be used at least once a day, preferably before retiring each night. Just slip the floss between two teeth and rake up and down each side of each tooth several times. When the tooth surface is clean, the floss will squeak.

Unless your teeth fit together so tightly that you must use waxed floss, it's best to use *unwaxed* floss. Some people prefer to use waxed dental *tape* to avoid injury to sensitive gums. But remember that unwaxed *floss* is best for raking away hardened deposits. You can avoid injury to your gums by working floss or tape between your teeth with a sawing motion so that it doesn't suddenly snap against your gum. The next time you have your teeth cleaned, ask the dentist or hygienist to show you how to use dental floss.

Note: It takes about 24 hours for plaque (which may be invisible) to build up on the teeth. This plaque can be easily removed by using dental floss once a day along with brushing. If plaque is allowed to remain on the teeth longer than 24 hours, however, it begins to harden and is more difficult to remove. Be sure to take your floss with you when you go on a trip.

CLEAN GUM POCKETS
WITH ORAL IRRIGATION

Once gum pockets develop, it's practically impossible to clean them without using an oral irrigation device. This is a small water pump that you can use to direct a pressurized, pulsating stream of water up under gum margins. You can wash all kinds of garbage from gum pockets, even after you brush your teeth and rake them with dental floss. Try it and see. Proper use of an oral irrigation device, especially after the age of 40, can mean the difference between keeping your teeth or losing them. You can purchase an oral irrigation device in any drug store for about $25.

Persons with gum disease should irrigate their gums after each meal to remove food particles from gum pockets and to wash away bacteria. Decayed matter in gum pockets can cause very bad breath, and the longer this matter remains in deep pockets the worse your breath will be. If you wake up each morning with bad breath in spite of brushing your teeth the night before, chances are there is food residue under the edges of your gums. If there is a bacterial infection in gum pockets, you'll have to use oral irrigation morning, noon, and night to keep your breath fresh.

When food particles remain in the gum pockets longer than 24 hours, bacterial activity may produce the kind of breath that smells like the food residue in your colon! No celebrity can afford such breath. You can't either, if you want to be close to people. You can test your breath for odor by placing a clean glass over your mouth and nose and sniffing the air you exhale into the glass.

Note: The fleshy fuzz covering your tongue can catch food particles that may decompose and cause bad breath. So be sure to brush your tongue occasionally, especially if it appears to be coated.

SMILE!

If you have good teeth, you should proudly show off your teeth every chance you get by smiling. In addition to making you more attractive, a smile is so contagious that its effect on others will be returned to you with genuine warmth. When we asked ever-smiling *Gavin MacLeod* (the skipper of the "Love Boat") if he did anything special for his teeth, he replied: "I brush my teeth constantly! I'm always brushing my teeth. Especially *now* because the women are now saying 'Oh, man, I love your smile.' I want to keep that smile looking *good.*"

Remember that bad teeth make it difficult to smile. They can also shatter the aura of your physical appeal when you open your mouth. Make sure that care of your teeth is a part of your body program. And keep smiling!

DON'T NEGLECT YOUR NAILS

In the animal kingdom, teeth and nails often serve as weapons; hence the fighting expression "Coming at you tooth and nail." We humans, however, use our teeth only in eating and in articulating speech, and we use our nails primarily to scratch itchy skin. We also groom our teeth and nails to improve our sex appeal. Our nails are a little more than adornments that add to the beauty of our hands and feet.

Poorly groomed nails detract greatly from your physical appearance. Dirty nails certainly reflect upon your personal cleanliness. Your teeth and your skin may deserve more attention than your nails, but you certainly should not neglect your nails. "It doesn't make sense to wear gorgeous clothes and then have ugly hands," advises *Cher Bono*. "Your nails are really part of your outfit."

Beautify your Nails with Food

Your teeth are formed primarily from calcium, but your nails are made of protein. This means that your nails, like your skin must be constantly nourished with a good diet or they'll rapidly deteriorate. Lack of adequate protein, for example, will result in thin, weak nails that break easily. A great many nutrients are involved in the formation of a nail, however, so be sure to eat a balanced diet of fresh, natural foods.

Some doctors believe that eating gelatin helps harden brittle nails. But since gelatin is not a complete protein, it must be used in conjunction with other foods that supply protein. If you do supplement your diet with gelatin, mix about one-fourth of an ounce of unflavored gelatin into a glass of orange juice.

Remember that detergents, cleaners, nail polish removers, and other products applied to the nails can make nails brittle. There are a great many diseases that deform nails. Anemia, for example, can affect the shape of your nails. A fungus infection can result in rough, lumpy nails, and so on. Be sure to check with your doctor if your nails appear to be abnormal.

The late *Adelle Davis* recommended protein and Vitamin A for abnormal nails. If fungus infection was present, she recommended large doses of Vitamin B. "When a diet has been grossly inadequate," she observed, "large amounts of B vitamins must be obtained for a prolonged period before some fungus infestations, like those around the fingernails, clear up."

HOW TO GROOM YOUR NAILS

Dirt under the nails is best removed by first soaking them in soapy water before scraping away the dirt with a plastic or wooden strip. Don't ever scrape your nails with a metallic object. Tiny scratches left on the underside of a nail will accumulate dirt that is difficult or impossible to remove.

Nails should be clipped *after* they have been softened by a warm bath. Cuticles softened by washing can be pushed back with an orange stick. Wait until your nails are *dry* before filing them. Use a fine *emery board* rather than a metal file. Bevel the edges of your nails by filing at a 45-degree angle. Use the file to knock off sharp corners on each side of the nail. Hangnails should be snipped off with clippers.

If you have a problem with hangnails or brittle nails, your nails might be suffering from excessive dryness. You know from reading Chapter 5 that keeping your hands in water promotes dryness by dissolving protective oils. Wear cotton-lined rubber gloves when washing clothes, dishes, windows, or the family car. Occasionally soak your hands in cool water for a few minutes, pat them dry, and then rub them with vegetable oil to hold in the absorbed moisture. Keep your nails cut as short as possible to minimize splitting and peeling, to prevent breaking, and to facilitate cleaning.

In Hollywood at the present time, *long* nails are fasionable. Long or short, "Beautiful nails are really high status at the moment," reports Beverly Hills manicurist *Nina Rico.* "They are a sign of wealth and good breeding."

WHAT ABOUT TOENAILS?

You care for your toenails much the same way you care for fingernails—except that you *always cut toenails short.* Be careful not to wear shoes that squeeze your toes together. Constant pressure on toenails can result in ingrown nails or even loss of a nail.

When you clip toenails, cut the nails so that they are only slightly rounded and then file off sharp corners. Be careful not to cut the nails too far back at the corners. Let the nail protrude far enough on each side to make sure that the corners of the nail are not covered by skin. If the nail is cut back so far that the corners of the nail are not visible, the pressure placed upon them by shoes may press the nail corners into the flesh. Most ingrown toenails are the result of squeezing the toes with tight shoes.

No matter how carefully you groom your toenails, make sure that your shoes are long enough and wide enough to give your toes plenty of room.

SUMMARY

1. You must have good teeth to chew a variety of natural foods if you want a healthy body.

2. Tooth decay is caused primarily by bacteria that live off the sugar and refined carbohydrates in your diet.

3. More teeth are lost to gum disease than to all other factors combined.

4. Try to eliminate the sugar and white-flour products in your diet and then brush your teeth after each meal.

5. Unwaxed dental floss used once every 24 hours will rake plaque and other deposits off your teeth.

6. An oral irrigation device that directs a pulsating stream of water up under your gum margins can be used after each meal to wash food particles from gum pockets.

7. If you have bad breath and bleeding gums in spite of taking good care of your teeth, make an appointment with a periodontist.

8. Just as good nutrition is important to the formation of a healthy tooth, you must continue to eat properly to maintain healthy gums and strong nails.

9. Don't fail to groom your nails if you want to keep your body attractive and appealing.

10. Toenails should be cut fairly straight across so that the corners of the nail are not covered by flesh.

7

The Celebrity Approach to Handling Body Aches and Pains at Home

No matter how well you take care of your health, you're going to suffer an occasional body ache or pain as a result of strain or injury. Backache, for example, while commonly caused by weak muscles and poor posture, can result from improper lifting techniques and other factors that can injure the strongest of backs. Headache can result from additives in the food you eat as well as from stress and tension. It's practically impossible to avoid a little trouble with arthritis, tendonitis, and other mechanical problems as you grow older.

How you care for your aches and pains at home will have much to do with whether they become major or minor problems. A simple back injury, for example, if improperly handled, can result in incapacitating disability. You should, of course, see your doctor when you suffer a serious injury or when pain persists unrelieved. But what you do to help yourself can make the difference between rapid and complete recovery or chronic disability.

Every celebrity who must meet a rigid working or personal-appearance schedule is aware of the value of self-help in caring for ailments that could result in cancellation of an important or lucrative engagement. If you have a family, the old show business adage "The show must go on" applies as much to you as it does to a celebrity. The show must go on for you, too, if you want to enjoy life and continue bringing home a paycheck. Even if you are strong and healthy, study this chapter carefully so that you'll know what to do to *prevent* body aches and pains as well as what to do when they occur.

As the host of a daily television game show, vivacious *Ruta Lee* must stay healthy and strong to keep up her pace and to inspire guests. To do this, she takes the best possible care of herself—as you should do if you want to live fully and work hard.

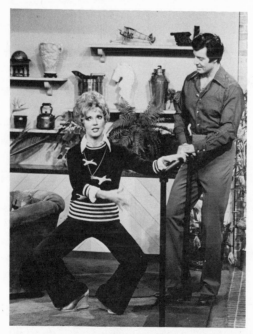

Ruta Lee, hostess of NBC's "High Rollers" television show, prevents aches and pains by doing stretching exercises with a stationary bar.

BACKACHE: THE NO. 1 AILMENT

In 1975, according to the U.S. Department of Health, Education and Welfare, *back trouble was the most common complaint of people who visited family doctors or general practitioners.* Nothing is more incapacitating than back trouble. Even a minor injury to the lower back can make it impossible to work or play.

Because of the tremendous amount of pressure and leverage placed on the joints and discs of the spine in everyday activities, the pain and disability resulting from an injury to the lower portion of the spine are usually out of proportion to the seriousness of the injury. So don't panic if you can't get out of bed the morning after hurting your back. Chances are that after a few days the acuteness of the injury will subside and you'll gradually get back to normal. There are, however, some basic procedures that you should follow in caring for your back. And there are danger signals that you should watch for in case you need medical care.

It's Usually Only a Strain

Lumbosacral strain is the most common cause of back pain. The lumbosacral joints are located at the bottom of the spine where the lower back joins the pelvis. Most of the time, a low-back strain occurs as a result of a postural strain or an improper lifting technique. Pain and disability may be immediate—or they may gradually develop overnight following a slight injury that initially caused only a twinge of pain. The reason for this delayed reaction is that there is a gradual and progressive swelling in the injured tissues.

Choosing Between
Cold Packs and Hot Packs

When an injury to the back results in immediate pain and disability, it might be a good idea to apply a cold pack for half an hour every two or three hours during the first day. The cold will constrict blood vessels and cut down on the amount of swelling in the injured tissues. You can make a cold pack by putting ice cubes into a plastic ziplock bag which may then be wrapped or laid over a damp towel. After 24 hours or so, you may begin to apply moist heat.

When a back injury has a delayed reaction and does not result in pain or disability until the next day, you may begin treatment with moist heat, even if you did not use cold the day before. Most injuries that are severe enough to require cold applications will result in *immediate* pain.

How to Make a
Steaming-Hot Fomentation

You can make an effective fomentation or moist heat pack simply by laying a hot water bottle or an insulated heating pad over a damp towel. Or you may direct the rays of an infrared lamp down onto a damp towel that has been laid over the injured area. If you don't have any heating devices, you may simply wring a towel out in hot water and then wrap it in flannel to hold in heat and moisture. Here's the procedure we recommend:

1. Place a large piece of dry flannel over the injured portion of the back.
2. Fold a large towel into a 12-inch square.
3. Roll up the towel and soak it in hot water; then wring it out until it's no longer dripping.
4. Unroll the towel on top of the flannel-covered back and then fold the edges of the flannel over the towel to seal in the heat.
5. Repeat the application when it cools. Do this at least three times. Each time the application is changed, dry the skin and use a fresh piece of dry flannel.

Play It Safe with Rest

Rest is always indicated when a back injury is painful. Resting doesn't necessarily mean that you must stay in bed. You should, of course, rest in bed when movement is painful. But it's occasionally best to move around a little to prevent excessive stiffness. Be guided by the way you feel. If pain is relieved by bed rest, then stay in bed until you feel better. If bed rest seems to make you feel worse, then do what you feel best doing. The important thing is to *avoid doing anything that seems to aggravate your back.* Don't get yourself into a situation where you cannot lie down if you feel the need to do so. Avoid chores or activities that seem to increase your discomfort or put a strain on your back. Taking a few days off from work may be all you need to do to rest your back, even if you don't go to bed.

When comedienne *Charlotte Rae* appeared as a guest on "Peter Lupus' Body Shop" television show, she was literally down in her back. She had to be propped up with pillows during her interview. While she was on camera in the studio kitchen, she nearly fell to the floor when her knees buckled from a back spasm. With the indomitable spirit of a seasoned performer, however, the courageous comedienne completed the filming of the show before leaving for home. Charlotte confessed that her back trouble had started many weeks earlier, but a busy schedule had not permitted any time for rest. "It wasn't bad to begin with," she said, "but I aggravated it by working long hours."

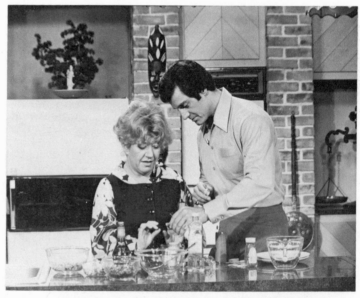

*TV comedienne Charlotte Rae, co-star of "Diff'rent
Strokes," is so health conscious that she uses all-natural
methods in the care of her aches and pains.*

We advised Charlotte to go home and *rest* and to begin using moist heat applications. After a short time, she was back at work filming her new television series "Facts of Life."

Remember that it's always best to give your back the benefit of a doubt and rest when activity causes pain. You cannot get rid of a back pain by "working it off" if the work you do makes the pain worse.

Sleep on a Firm Bed

Everyone should sleep on a firm bed. When you're having back trouble, a firm bed is essential. But don't make your bed *too* hard. Ideally, your bed should be firm enough to prevent sagging of your spine but soft enough to mold itself to the contours of your body. If you feel that your mattress sags, you can place a half-inch thick sheet of plywood between the mattress and the springs—or you may simply place your mattress on the floor. If you use a sheet of plywood, be sure to cut the wood so that its dimensions are a little less than those of the mattress. And round the corners so that there won't be any sharp protrusions.

"Until I started sleeping on a firm mattress, I used to get up every morning with a backache," Jim W. testified. "That one simple measure eliminated a backache that had persisted unrelieved for 10 years!"

Actor *Peter Lawford* has chronic back trouble that is aggravated by a sagging mattress and relieved by using a bed board. "When I go to a hotel, especially in New York where the mattresses are usually soft, the first thing I ask for is a board," Peter divulged. "Once, in another country, I asked for a board and they brought me a *door!* It didn't have a knob or anything on it, but it was an old door. It helped, though. It was better than nothing."

A mattress that is *too hard* can be softened by covering it with a thick sheet of foam rubber. It's all right to sleep on a fairly soft mattress if it does not sag in the middle.

The best way to sleep when you're having back trouble is to lie flat on your back with a pillow under your knees. Lying with your knees slightly bent will prevent painful arching of your lower back and allow your back muscles to relax. It might be all right to sleep on your side if you find that you can do so comfortably, but it's never a good idea to sleep on your stomach.

Watch for Danger Signals

Most of the time, a low-back strain will respond to heat, rest, time, a firm mattress, and other simple measures. Your body does a marvelous job of healing itself. But when back trouble persists longer than a couple of weeks, or if there is considerable pain or any unusual symptoms, you should see a doctor. *Gavin MacLeod* of "Love Boat" suffered from chronic backache until he finally got professional help. "And you know what the problem was? It was from a broken bone in my foot!" he exclaimed. "Everything is really connected, as you know. And now what's happening is my chiropractor is building something for my shoe. I have something in my shoe right now, as a matter of fact. It affects my walk, my hip, and everything else. Until I found out what was wrong, I had a miserable kind of thing. Since I've been wearing this pad in my shoe my back has been perfect."

You should seek professional help, too, if home care does not relieve your backache.

HOW TO DISTINGUISH KIDNEY TROUBLE FROM BACK TROUBLE

Any time you have a backache that is accompanied by fever, you might have an infection that requires medical care. A kidney infection, for example, commonly causes backache. The only way you can diagnose a kidney infection is to have your urine examined by a doctor. There are, however, a few simple ways to distinguish back trouble from a possible kidney infection.

If you have pain that is aggravated by movement, that is, if it hurts your back to bend, sneeze, get out of your car, or turn over in bed, your trouble is obviously mechanical in nature. And if your back trouble started with a fall, an awkward movement, or while lifting an object, no one will have to tell you that you have injured your back. When you have a backache that is *not* aggravated by movement, the backache may then be a symptom of some other disorder. A kidney infection should always be suspected when you have a fever and you do not feel well. *If you have a fever, or if you have a backache that is not affected by moving or bending, see your doctor for a checkup.*

WHAT TO DO ABOUT A SLIPPED DISC

Low-back trouble resulting from a simple strain is not often serious. But when it is accompanied by aching, numbness, or tingling that radiates into your thigh, calf, or foot, you might be having trouble with a disc.

Intervertebral discs are thick cartilage cushions that separate the vertebrae and serve as shock absorbers. When one of these discs ruptures, it often bulges out and hits a nerve that supplies skin and muscles in a portion of the leg. This results in symptoms only in the part of the leg supplied by the nerve. A doctor can usually tell which disc is involved by the location of the symptoms. A ruptured disc must occasionally be removed surgically to prevent nerve damage.

There are many causes of leg pain, including tumors and blood clots. You should *always* be examined by a doctor when you have leg pain of unknown origin.

Stretch Your Back at Home

Once a diagnosis of slipped (herniated) disc has been made, you might be able to help yourself (and avoid surgery) by using a traction rig at home to stretch your spine. Ask your doctor about using traction. Any surgical supply store can furnish you with a traction apparatus, complete with detailed instructions on how to use it.

Supplement your diet with B complex vitamins to speed healing of damaged nerve fibers. Take up to 2,000 milligrams of Vitamin C in daily divided doses to strengthen the collagen in weak disc fibers. Zinc and manganese are also often prescribed.

A good chiropractor or osteopath can stretch the spine with manipulative techniques that are designed to expand discs and loosen vertebrae. *Paul Lynde* of "Hollywood Squares" depends upon chiropractors in caring for a chronic back problem. "I have a bad back and chiropractors give me relief," he says. "If that one bone in your spine is out, there's flesh in there being pinched. And if you don't get the bone put back right, it's going to go right on pinching that flesh."

Avoid Drugs Whenever Possible

Leg pain caused by a herniated disc is occasionally severe

Comedian *Bob Hope* keeps his disc problem under control by taking vitamins, hanging from Roman rings, and getting regular massages. "The rings are the greatest thing in the world," he maintains. "I have them outside my Palm Springs home where I hang for a minute to a minute and a half and just stretch a little. If you ever get back trouble, try that."

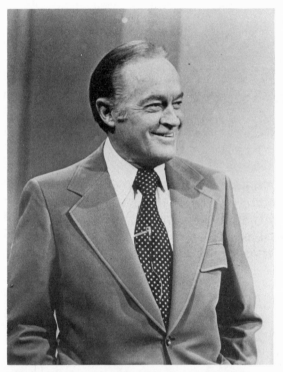

Comedian Bob Hope treats his back trouble with a spinal stretching exercise that he does at home.

enough to require the use of pain-killing drugs. You should avoid the use of drugs whenever possible, however. Once it has been established that your leg pain is not serious and you can tolerate the pain, you should continue with home treatment and try to live with the pain—provided, of course, that you keep in touch with your doctor.

Ricardo Montalban, of TV's "Fantasy Island," has endured 20 years of leg pain caused by nerve damage when he was thrown from a horse. "The sensory nerves in my right leg were damaged," he explained, "so I have no feeling of hot or cold in that leg. The motor nerves were also injured, leaving the leg partially paralyzed . ... But I have grown to live with it and the constant pain." Montalban does not depend upon drugs to relieve his pain. "Drugs can dull the brain," he warns, "and that is something, as an actor, I can't have. I would rather have the pain than risk giving up control of my faculties."

We all know what happened to former First Lady *Betty Ford* when she relied upon the use of drugs to relieve the pain of a pinched neck nerve. After 13 years of chronic pain, she had to undergo treatment for drug addiction! Comedian *Jerry Lewis* admitted recently that he once contemplated suicide after 13 years of addiction to a drug he took to relieve back pain. Finally freed from his addiction he told reporters that he felt "cleansed and reborn."

When you have a chronic back ailment, try some of the treatment methods described in this chapter before resorting to the use of drugs. Simple aspirin is often just as effective as a prescription drug in relieving pain—and it's safer. Aspirin should be used only on a short-term basis, however. Excessive use of aspirin can inflame your stomach, interfere with normal clotting of blood, force elimination of Vitamin C from your body, and occasionally result in dizziness and other side effects.

EXERCISES FOR A
STRONG AND HEALTHY BACK

When *Dr. Samuel Homola* appeared on "Peter Lupus' Body Shop," he demonstrated two exercises that he felt were adequate for strengthening a weak back. "Picture the muscles surrounding your spine as guy wires on a TV antenna," he told television viewers, "and you can understand why you must have strong supporting muscles on both sides of your spine. You can strengthen these muscles with two simple exercises."

Here are the two exercises demonstrated by Dr. Homola and actress *Alexis Alexander* on the show.

Exercise 1: The Bent-Knee
Leg Lift and Trunk Curl

Lie on your back with your knees bent and your arms alongside your body. Hold your knees in a bent position while you lift your knees up toward your chest. Contract your abdominal muscles and curl your trunk so that you lift your hips from the floor. (See the photo.)

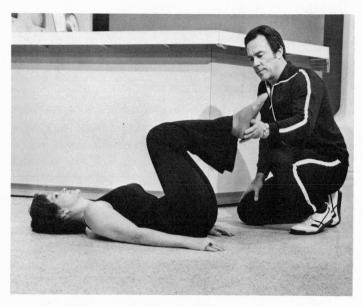

Actress Helen Schuh receives instruction from Dr. Samuel Homola in performing her bent-knee leg lifts that are designed to strengthen back-supporting hip flexors.

This exercise will strengthen the abdominal muscles and hip flexors that serve as "guy wires" on the *front side* of your spine. Begin with only a few repetitions and work your way up to about 15 repetitions over a period of time. Exhale while lifting your legs.

Exercise 2: The Progressive
Back-Arching Exercise

To strengthen the muscles on the *back side* of your spine, place a sofa cushion on the floor and lie face down over the cushion so that it supports your pelvic and abdominal areas. Place your feet under the edge of a heavy sofa or have someone hold your feet down. Arch your upper body up from the floor without using your arms. (See the photo.) As your back becomes stronger, you can move the cushion down for greater leverage. Begin with only a few repetitions and work your way up to 10 or more. Do not try to arch up as high as you can. Keep the exercise comfortable by avoiding forceful or maximum contraction of your back muscles lest you suffer a painful cramp.

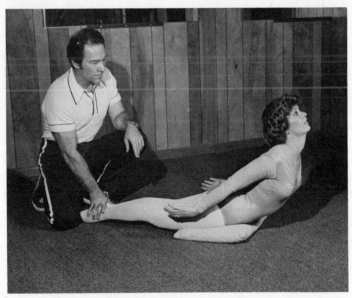

*Model Kim Ashbrook performs a back-arching exercise
that strengthens weak back muscles.*

Actor *Lyle Waggoner* described a leg bicep exercise that he believes cured his disc problem (see Chapter 11). The exercise is performed by lying face down and curling both legs against resistance. Most gyms and spas have a leg-curl machine.

Robert Pine of "Chips" keeps his back problem under control by exercising. "As long as I'm exercising," he says, "my back doesn't bother me. If I stop exercising, almost two to three weeks after that, my back goes out automatically. But I find that if I exercise *regularly* I don't have any back trouble at all."

HOW TO KEEP GOING
WITH ARTHRITIS

Arthritis ranks high on the list of chronic cripplers, and it is no respecter of persons. *Dr. Christian Bernard,* the first doctor to do a heart transplant, suffers from arthritis. Rich or poor, famous or unknown, you may be just as susceptible to arthritis as the next person. Estimates on the number of people suffering from arthritis range from 16 million to 66 million. No one really knows what causes arthritis, but hereditary predisposition and diet are believed to be underlying factors.

According to *Dr. Edith Weir* of the U.S. Department of Agriculture, "All of the arthritic conditions appear to be associated with adverse changes in nutrient metabolism." The specific dietary changes needed to prevent the development of arthritis are not known, but it makes good sense to eat a balanced diet of fresh, natural foods in preventing as well as in treating arthritis. Once arthritis develops, there are a few specific measures that should be taken to control the disease and prevent crippling. Osteoarthritis, rheumatoid arthritis, and gout are the most common forms of arthritis. What you do to help yourself depends upon the type of arthritis you have. If your doctor tells you that you have arthritis, ask him to be more specific.

How to Handle Osteoarthritis

Osteoarthritis is caused primarily by injury or wear and tear on joints. When your joints begin to stiffen from osteoarthritis, usually after the age of 40, it's important to get enough exercise to maintain your mobility but not so much that you inflame your joints. Simple moist heat, such as that recommended earlier for back trouble, applied over the affected joints will usually relieve the pain. When all of the joints of the body are affected, soaking in a tub of hot water, followed by movement of all the joints through a full range of movement, will be beneficial.

Supplement a balanced diet of natural foods with at least 500 milligrams of Vitamin C to help rebuild worn joint cartilage. And make sure that you get at least 1,000 milligrams of calcium and 400 units of Vitamin D each day to maintain the strength of your bones. Taking a betaine hydrochloride tablet with meals may assure more efficient absorption of calcium in older persons. Vitamin B complex will increase metabolic efficiency.

Note: Taking calcium will *not* add to the calcium deposits in arthritis. Calcium spurs that build up around joints are the result of chronic irritation and have nothing to do with the amount of calcium in your diet. If your diet is deficient in calcium, your body will simply take calcium from your bones to form arthritic spurs, thus weakening your bones and making joints more susceptible to arthritis. So even if you do have "calcium spurs," you must make sure that your diet contains adequate calcium to keep your bones strong and hard in combating the effects of arthritis.

How to Relieve Rheumatoid Arthritis

Rheumatoid arthritis is the most crippling form of arthritis, and it usually begins before the age of 40. Most doctors believe that rheumatoid arthritis is a systemic or metabolic disorder that affects all of the connective tissues of the body.

It's absolutely essential that persons suffering from rheumatoid arthritis eat only fresh, natural foods with adequate protein and calcium. It might be helpful to supplement the diet with such concentrated natural food substances as brewer's yeast, desiccated liver, bone meal, and wheat germ along with essential vitamins and minerals. Pyridoxine (Vitamin B_6) and pantothenic acid in doses up to 100 milligrams a day may improve metabolic efficiency. Many arthritic patients who take such supplements report an improvement in their condition. "Since I've been taking the vitamins and supplements you prescribed," said 38-year-old Wanda D., "my arthritis has improved tremendously!"

Exercise is important, but fatigue should be avoided. Freedom from mental and emotional stress is essential. Whatever you do, avoid processed foods containing sugar, white flour, preservatives, and artificial additives.

How to Control Gouty Arthritis

Contrary to popular belief, you don't have to live "high on the hog" or eat rich foods to develop gout. You can inherit susceptibility to gout. This means that your body cannot adequately metabolize the purines supplied by meats, beans, and certain other purine-rich foods. The result is that uric acid (a by-product of purine metabolism) tends to accumulate in your joints. The effect of uric acid in a joint is like placing ground glass between sensitive joint surfaces.

If you don't already have gout, don't worry about your diet. You should go right ahead and eat meats, beans, and other natural foods in a balanced diet. You won't develop gout, no matter what you eat, if you don't have the metabolic disorder that predisposes you to gout. If you *do* develop a swollen, painful joint (most often in the foot) and a blood test reveals an abnormally high level of uric acid, you might have to eliminate a few otherwise healthful foods from your diet.

There are certain drugs that can be used to control gout while you continue to eat anything you want. In severe cases, it's often necessary to use such drugs. But you should first try to control gout with dietary measures. If you can prevent the development of painful joints by eliminating purine-rich foods from your diet, it would be better to use dietary measures than to depend upon potentially harmful drugs. Use the celebrity approach and try our dietary recommendations before resorting to regular use of drugs. Use drugs only to relieve acute attacks of gouty arthritis and then see if changing your diet will prevent recurring attacks. If it turns out that your body is *manufacturing* an excessive amount of uric acid, you may have to take regular medication in spite of altering your diet.

Note: Persons who go on a crash diet and lose a large amount of weight may develop a *temporary* case of gouty arthritis. A rapid breaking down of body tissues may release more uric acid than the body can eliminate at one time. Try to avoid losing more than two or three pounds a week if you want to avoid trouble. If you have weight to lose, follow the program we recommend in Chapter 1.

A Diet to Relieve Gouty Arthritis

If you have gouty arthritis, you should avoid these purine-rich foods: Sweetbreads (animal pancreas and thymus), sardines, anchovies, kidney, liver, brain, meat, meat extracts, gravies, fish, game, fowl, beans, lentils, spices, condiments, and alcoholic beverages.

You can get adequate purine-free protein from nuts, seeds, skimmed milk, eggs, cheese, cottage cheese, and protein supplements.

Whole-grain wheat contains a moderate amount of purine. Try to eat corn bread rather than wheat bread. Whole-grain cereals can be replaced by grits and cream of wheat.

Wheat germ, desiccated liver, and brewer's yeast also contain purine. You may have to go easy on the use of these supplements if you use dietary measures to control gouty arthritis.

Eat plenty of fresh fruits and vegetables. Drink up to three quarts of liquids a day to aid your kidneys in eliminating uric acid. Fruit and vegetable juices will help combat the formation of uric acid kidney stones by alkalizing your urine. Avoid beverages containing caffeine (coffee, tea, cocoa, and colas).

Since ascorbic acid (Vitamin C) tends to acidify the urine and form oxalates in the body, you might have to be cautious about taking large doses of any form of Vitamin C if you have gouty arthritis. (Calcium oxalate stones, like uric acid stones, form in acid urine.) It does not take much ascorbic acid to acidify the urine, but it may take more than 4,000 milligrams of Vitamin C daily to result in significant increases in urine oxalate.

EMERGENCY TREATMENT
FOR TENSION HEADACHE

When we were filming "Peter Lupus' Body Shop" television series, we filmed five half-hour shows a day. This resulted in a great deal of tension for everyone involved and caused many tension headaches. During Dr. Samuel Homola's appearance on show No. 84, he demonstrated a neck adjustment on actress Alexis Alexander. "This is great for relieving tension headaches," he said while tugging on her neck. Everyone on the set must have had a headache. After the show, the entire crew lined up for a neck adjustment!

If you suffer from tension headaches, there is a simple way to "adjust" your neck at home. You can use the same technique we recommend for people on the go. You'll have to have a little help, however, so find a partner who can follow instructions in applying the treatment to your neck.

"When I'm traveling and I develop a tension headache," say Randy V., a sales representative, "I have my partner use your metho on my neck. It always relieves my headache. Sometimes I can get a airline stewardess to do it for me after I show her how to do it."

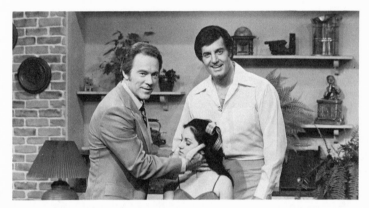

*Dr. Samuel Homola demonstrates a tension-relieving,
neck-stretching adjustment on actress Alexis Alexander.*

How to Stretch Away Neck Tension

Simple tension, or prolonged contraction of the muscles on th back of the neck, is the most common cause of headache. In fac about seven out of ten headaches are caused by tension. This mean that in many cases you can relieve a headache by massaging an stretching the muscles on the back of the neck.

When a muscle is tight or in spasm, stretching the muscle wi usually force it to relax. The stretching will be more effective, howeve if it is preceded by a little massage to stimulate blood flow. Demor strate the following massage and stretching techniques to a partne before having him use them on you.

Massage technique: Have your partner sit on a low stool or on dining room chair. Then place your left hand (if you're right handec on his forehead so that you can support his head when he tilts

ɔrward. It's very important for your partner to let his head rest against
ʝour hand so that the muscles on the back of his neck are completely
ȝelaxed.

Encircle the back of his neck (at the base of his skull) with the
ɪumb and forefinger of your right hand. Massage the neck muscles
ʳhere they attach to the skull by moving the massaging hand up and
ɪown in a tight circular motion. Be sure to press the massaging hand
ʳrmly against the neck so that it will stay in contact with the skin as it
ɪdes over the muscles. Don't let your hand slide over the skin to
ʳreate an uncomfortable friction. About 30 seconds of neck massage
ʝill flush muscle attachments with a fresh flow of blood and get rid of
ʳritating waste products.

Stretching technique: The neck muscles should be stretched
ɪmmediately after they have been massaged. If your partner is sitting
ɪ a chair, have him turn 90 degrees so that he is sitting "side saddle"
ɪ an erect position. Stand behind him and place the forepart of your
ɪght foot (your left foot if you are left handed) up on the edge of the
ɪhair seat. Cup your hands around the base of his skull and his jaws
ɪn each side and rest your right elbow on your right knee.

Lift your partner's head (to stretch his neck muscles) by pulling
ʝith your hands and raising the heel of the foot that's up on the chair.
ȝe sure to keep your wrists rigid so that movement of the supporting
ɪnee will aid your arms in lifting the head. Exert a slow, steady pull
ɪntil the neck is fully stretched and then slowly release the pull. Repeat
ɪnd stretch at least three times. Alternately stretching and releasing
ɪght neck muscles (intermittent traction) is the best way known to
ɪelieve neck tension.

Once you have demonstrated the massaging and stretching
ȝechniques to a partner, have him perform them on you. Make sure
ɪhat you *sit as erect as possible* so that the stretching will be specific
ɔr your neck muscles.

Iome Head Harness

If you suffer from chronic neck tension and headaches, you
ɪight want to purchase a cervical traction apparatus for use at home.
ʰhis is a head harness equipped with weights, a cord, and a pulley that
ʳan be used to place a continuous pull on your neck. You can apply

the traction while sitting in a doorway or while lying in bed. Any surgical supply store can issue traction equipment and show you how to use it, but it must be prescribed by a physician.

Miscellaneous Headache Remedies

Simple, moist heat applied to the muscles on the back of the neck is a good way to relax tight neck muscles, especially when the muscles have been inflamed by chronic tension. A vascular headache can sometimes be relieved by placing an ice pack on the head or on the front of the neck to constrict swollen blood vessels. The caffeine supplied by a strong cup of coffee also constricts blood vessels. This is why aspirin and other headache remedies are often combined with caffeine. Remember, however, that caffeine, like sugar and white-flour products, can trigger hypoglycemia in some people, which can result in a headache. Sodium nitrates, nitrites, monosodium glutamate, salt and other additives in processed or preserved foods commonly result in a vascular headache. Nitrites, for example, are often used medically to dilate blood vessels. Eating foods preserved or colored with nitrites can result in a rapid pulse, flushing of the face, and a throbbing headache caused by dilation of the blood vessels. The only remedy for this type of headache is to avoid eating artificially preserved foods.

There are, of course, many causes of headaches, and some can be serious or even fatal. If you experience a painful or persistent headache, or if you have a headache that is accompanied by fever, vomiting, visual disturbances, or any other unusual symptoms, be sure to see your doctor.

HOW TO HANDLE STRAINS AND SPRAINS

A wrist, knee, or ankle sprain can occur unexpectedly at the most inopportune time. How you handle the injury during the first 24 hours can make the difference between prolonged disability or a rapid recovery. An ankle sprain is the most common injury and is often the most incapacitating. Every joint sprain should receive the same basic treatment. So whether you sprain your wrist, elbow, knee, or ankle, you should follow these basic procedures step by step in caring for the injury.

Step 1: Apply a Cold Pack Immediately

No matter where you are, on a Hollywood set, on an athletic field, or in your home, you should apply a cold pack to an injured joint as soon as possible. Cold will constrict the blood vessels in the injured tissues and reduce bleeding and swelling.

You can make an effective cold pack by filling a plastic ziploc bag with crushed ice and then wrapping it in a moist towel. Apply the cold pack over the injured joint for 20 to 30 minutes every two hours.

If you immerse a sprained ankle in a pan of water, add enough ice cubes to cool the water to a temperature of 50 to 60 degrees Fahrenheit. Remember, however, that you should keep a freshly sprained ankle elevated as much as possible. So it's usually best to apply an ice pack to your ankle while you're lying down.

In the case of an elbow sprain, athletes often slip a section of an automobile inner tube over the arm before immersing the elbow in a bucket of water. This protects the skin from damaging contact with the ice and distributes the cold evenly.

Cold should be applied to a sprained joint off and on for 24 to 48 hours, depending upon how bad the sprain is. Even if you do not use cold, you should wait at least 48 hours before applying heat. Applied too soon, heat will draw blood to the injured tissues and increase the swelling. When in doubt, apply cold.

Between applications of cold, wrap the injured joint with an elastic bandage. Keep the joint elevated as much as possible to reduce blood flow into the injured tissues.

Step 2: After 48 Hours, Apply Heat

After 48 hours, bleeding has usually stopped and swelling begins to subside, permitting the use of heat. If the application of heat causes throbbing pain, however, apply cold and wait 24 hours before trying heat again. Once the injured blood vessels have sealed themselves, heat will speed healing by stimulating blood flow and opening clogged arteries and veins. You may simply immerse the injured joint in comfortably hot water (about 105 degrees Fahrenheit) for 15 to 20 minutes two or three times a day or apply a hot compress (described earlier). In the case of the knee, you'd have to use a hot compress.

Step 3: Use a Contrast Bath

Badly sprained ankles tend to accumulate blood, tissue fluid, and other products that seep from injured joints, ligaments, and blood vessels. Circulation may be reduced or obstructed by compressed or clogged blood vessels. If the escaped tissue products are not removed and the blood vessels opened, the accumulated debris may harden and result in adhesions, chronic swelling, and permanent thickening of the ankle.

The best way to break down clots, open blood vessels, and get rid of debris is to use a contrast bath, or *alternate* the use of hot and cold applications. This will literally *pump* blood through the injured tissues by alternately dilating and contracting tiny blood vessels. You should wait four or five days before applying such treatment, however, in order to make sure that the injured blood vessels have adequately healed; otherwise, fresh bleeding may occur.

To use a contrast bath on an injured ankle, you may simply immerse the foot in comfortably hot water for three minutes and then in comfortably cold water for one minute. Immerse the foot at least five times, alternating the hot water and the cold water. Begin with hot water and end with hot water. Use the contrast bath at least twice a day—once in the morning and once in the evening. In the case of a joint that cannot be immersed in water, you may simply alternate hot packs and cold packs.

Step 4: Begin Exercising

After you have rested an injured joint for several days, begin making an effort to move it through a full range of motion. Be guided by the way you feel. Don't force movement when it is painful. If you begin exercising the joint early enough, and you exercise it regularly, you'll prevent the development of adhesions that might result in permanent crippling.

Remember that the body you have is the only one you'll ever have. It deserves the best care you can give it—for *your* sake. So take the next step in your body-improvement program and read Chapter 8.

SUMMARY

1. Helping yourself in the care of aches and pains will speed your recovery and lessen chances of disability.

2. Backache is the most common complaint heard in doctors' offices.

3. Rest and moist heat are effective in the treatment of most back injuries.

4. Leg pain, with or without backache, should be brought to the attention of a doctor.

5. Backache caused by kidney infection is usually accompanied by fever and other symptoms.

6. Exercises to strengthen your back should develop muscles on the front and back sides of your spine.

7. In order for you to help yourself in the care of your arthritis, your doctor must tell you *what type* of arthritis you have.

8. Tension headaches can often be relieved by massaging and stretching the muscles of the neck.

9. You should always apply cold to fresh sprains and wait at least 48 hours before applying heat.

10. Refined and processed foods containing additives and preservatives can contribute to the development of arthritis, headache, and other problems.

8

How Celebrities Fight Colds, Infections, and Other Common Ailments

You already know from reading Chapter 4 that six of the ten leading causes of death in the United States have been linked to our *diet*. This means that heart disease, cancer, hardened arteries, diabetes, and other degenerative diseases that kill most of us can be prevented! There are many common ailments, such as colds and constipation, that can be handled successfully at home. You should, of course, find yourself a good family doctor that you can depend upon for a correct diagnosis of your ailments, so that you can do what needs to be done to maintain or restore your health. When there is a serious infection, for example, you might need an antibiotic to fight off invading bacteria. Advanced degenerative diseases might have to be controlled with surgery or medication. Caring for your body and your health, however, is *your* responsibility. It's up to you to do all you can to *prevent* disease and to keep your body strong and healthy. Drugs should be used only when absolutely necessary. When ailments occur that can benefit from self-help procedures, you may be able to avoid the need for drastic therapy by helping yourself.

A doctor trained in preventive medicine can actually predict the development of disease by observing a person's living and eating habits. You can *prevent* these diseases by taking a wholistic approach to building good health. This means doing everything you can to improve your mental and physical health with *natural* methods. In advising celebrities in the care of their bodies, we always recommend a wholistic approach. And in the care of common ailments, we recommend drugless self-help procedures whenever possible. This eliminates any possibility that health will be damaged by the treatment. In the case of an elevated blood cholesterol, for example, doctors often prescribe anti-cholesterol drugs. But unless changes are made in the diet, no permanent changes for the better can be made to protect the heart and the arteries. Furthermore, prolonged use of drugs could have dangerous side effects. (In rare cases, regular use of drugs may be necessary to control blood cholesterol elevated by a genetic defect.)

When *Dr. Philip Blaiberg* died of a heart attack 19 months after undergoing his historic heart transplant, an autopsy revealed that the arteries in his new heart were clogged with fat and cholesterol. The same disease that closed the arteries in his first heart had attacked the arteries in his second heart because no changes had been made in his diet. Had Dr. Blaiberg been given advice on the use of diet and supplements to prevent the development of coronary atherosclerosis, he might be alive today!

To survive, you must eliminate the *cause* of the disease or ailment that is threatening your life or torturing you body. And that's something that you must do yourself.

HOW TO PROTECT YOUR HEART
BY CLEANING OUT YOUR ARTERIES

When biochemist *Dr. Richard Passwater* appeared as a guest on "Peter Lupus' Body Shop" television show, we learned many interesting things about nutrition and the heart. Dr. Passwater maintains in his book *Supernutrition for Healthy Hearts* (Dial Press, 1977), for example, that dietary cholesterol does not cause heart disease. The general consensus among medical men, however, is that a diet high in fat and cholesterol *does* contribute to the development of heart disease. "The fear of cholesterol caused by this misinformation," says Dr. Passwater, "often conditions people to eat unbalanced diets by avoiding eggs, whole milk, butter, and meat. The resulting dietary deficiencies can actually *cause* premature heart disease."

We (Peter Lupus and Dr. Homola) have always recommended a balanced diet of fresh, natural foods for good health. This includes consumption of eggs, lean meat, and other wholesome foods. We do recommend, however, that you reduce your intake of *fat* as much as possible. Fat is rich in calories and may contribute to the development of overweight or cancer if not to the development of cardiovascular disease. (When you reduce your intake of *animal* fat, you automatically reduce your intake of cholesterol.) Since vegetable oil is a fat, it must also be used sparingly in a balanced diet.

There are many factors that contribute to the development of atherosclerosis and heart disease. Cigarette smoking, lack of exercise, nutrient deficiencies in an unbalanced diet, drinking chlorinated water, excessive use of refined and processed foods, consumption of too much sugar and salt, and stress, for example, all play a part in the clogging of arteries. Be sure to study the material in Chapter 4 for guidance in sensible, everyday eating habits. In the meantime, follow our celebrity guidelines in developing a strong heart with clean arteries.

The complete story on the cause and cure of heart disease has not yet been told. But there is plenty that you can do *now* to protect yourself from heart disease, *the nation's No. 1 killer.* (According to the American Heart Association, diseases of the heart and blood vessels kill more Americans than all other causes of death combined.)

There are at least four steps that *you* must take to protect your heart.

Step 1: Watch Your Diet

If you don't already have heart disease or an excessive amount of fat or cholesterol in your blood, just concentrate on eating a balanced diet of fresh, natural foods (see Chapter 1). But make sure that you cut away the fat from the meat you eat—and don't use grease or oil in cooking. Remember that excessive use of refined carbohydrates (such as sugar and white-flour products) can deplete your body of chromium and B vitamins, increase the amount of triglycerides (fat) in your blood, and result in blood sugar problems, all of which contribute to the development of the vascular disease that leads to heart trouble.

If you are overweight or if you have a high level of fat or cholesterol in your blood, you may have to further reduce your intake of animal fat. (Don't forget that cholesterol is associated with animal fat.) Select the low-fat variety of such animal products as milk and cheese. Skimmed milk and cottage cheese, for example, are low in fat. The use of butter should be kept to a minimum, but it might be better to use butter rather than margarine. Consumption of egg yolk might have to be restricted until your blood cholesterol drops to a safe level. (Doctors consider cholesterol levels up to 250 milligrams per 100 milliliters of blood to be normal, but you should try to keep yours below 200. Triglycerides should not go above 100 milligrams percent.)

When you cut down on the amount of animal fat in your diet, you won't need more than one or two tablespoons of vegetable oil daily to balance the saturated (hard) and unsaturated (soft) fat in your diet. You may simply use a cold-pressed vegetable oil as a dressing on raw salads. Remember that excessive use of vegetable oil can lead to a Vitamin E deficiency that will allow oxidation of the oil to produce free radicals (rancidity) that might cause cancer as well as damage your arteries.

Step 2: Exercise Regularly

Regular exercise protects your heart by lowering abnormal blood levels of cholesterol and triglycerides and by opening blood vessels that supply the heart muscle. Endurance-type exercise, such as that recommended in Chapter 2, strengthens the heart muscle and results in the formation of high-density lipoproteins that keep cholesterol from penetrating arterial walls. Also, when your body has been conditioned by regular exercise, it will function more efficiently and require less oxygen, which will in turn relieve the workload on your heart.

Actor *Ed Asner,* who jogged to strengthen his heart and control his body weight, reported that regular jogging improved his blood pressure and minimized an irregular heart beat. "I first began jogging in my own backyard," he said. "I finally went out on the street to jog a couple of miles in the hills. I had to quit jogging about two months ago, however, because I developed a bone spur on my heel."

Comedian *Phil Foster* of "Laverne and Shirley" worked his way up to *five miles* of jogging after recovering from a heart problem. He started out by *walking* a mile a day and then gradually began jogging.

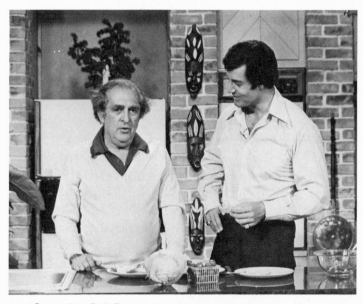

*Comedian Phil Foster of "Laverne and Shirley" regained
his health following a heart attack by exercising and
practicing good nutrition.*

Note: If you have heart trouble, you should exercise under the supervision of a physician.

Step 3: Supplement Your Diet
with Special Nutrients

There is a great deal of controversy surrounding the use of supplements in the treatment and prevention of heart disease. Some of us, however, feel that there is enough evidence supporting the value of supplements to warrant their use by anyone in *preventing* heart disease. Even if you eat a balanced diet, environmental factors and bad habits may drain nutrients from your body, making you more susceptible to heart disease. Air polluted with ozone consumes Vitamin E. The nicotine in cigarettes destroys Vitamin C in the blood. Sugar, alcohol, and birth control pills create a deficiency in the B vitamins, and so on.

We all know that Vitamin E is an important natural anticoagulant that helps prevent blood clots. The B vitamins, along with Vitamin C, lower blood cholesterol. Vitamin B_{15} (pangamate), found only in such natural foods as seeds, yeast, liver, and whole grains, increases the availability of oxygen in the blood and helps the heart utilize oxygen more efficiently. Lecithin, a substance extracted from soybeans, contains choline and other nutrients which are believed to lower blood cholesterol while increasing the level of protective high-density lipoproteins.

There are, of course, many other nutrients that are essential for clean arteries and a healthy heart. The minerals calcium, magnesium, and potassium, for example, must be supplied in a balanced diet. You must eat a variety of fresh, natural foods to be assured of getting all these nutrients. You should drink *hard* water for its calcium and magnesium content.

When you live under adverse conditions or do not eat properly, you should take supplements daily. Even a good diet must be supplemented when the body is diseased. Vitamin C and Vitamin E are probably the most important supplements to be used in conjunction with a balanced diet. Try working your way up to about 200 units of Vitamin E and 1,500 milligrams of Vitamin C daily in divided doses. Lecithin may be taken in tablet form or in granules. Lecithin granules can be added to health drinks and to foods. One or two tablespoons a day is the usual dosage.

Your body manufactures lecithin from elements supplied by a balanced diet. But when your blood cholesterol is elevated, or if there's any chance that your diet might be deficient in choline, Vitamin B_6, magnesium, essential fatty acids, and other nutrients your body needs to manufacture lecithin, it might be helpful to take lecithin in supplement form.

Brewer's yeast and wheat germ are good natural sources of the trace mineral selenium, an antioxidant that works with Vitamin E to help protect against heart disease.

Dr. Rinse's Breakfast Supplement

Some of our celebrity friends who are suffering from atherosclerosis are combining the use of lecithin and brewer's yeast in a mixture formulated by *Dr. Jacobus Rinse,* a physical chemist who reportedly used the mixture to cure his own heart disease. Dr. Rinse was first stricken with angina pectoris in 1951 at the age of 51. "Following the 1951 attack of angina pectoris with attendent violent heart aches," Dr. Rinse recalled, "the attending heart specialist predicted that I might have another 10 years to live if all physical exercise were avoided."

Dr. Rinse began a study of the cause of atherosclerosis and formulated a dietary supplement of his own. "Starting with an hypothesis that deficiencies in my food could be causative factors," he explained, "dietary changes were explored, resulting in the complete alleviation of angina and related heart diseases." Today, at the age of 78, Dr. Rinse is apparently free of heart disease.

Rinse's formula: To make Dr. Rinse's supplement, mix one tablespoon each of lecithin, yeast, and wheat germ with one teaspoon of bone meal. (You may, of course, mix a larger amount for storage, but stick to the suggested ratios.)

Take two tablespoons of the above mixture and mix with one tablespoon of dark brown sugar and one tablespoon of safflower oil (or some other vegetable oil).

Add milk to dissolve the sugar and yeast.

Add yogurt to increase consistency.

You may then add the completed mixture to hot or cold cereal, along with raisins and other fruits if desired. (*American Laboratory,* July, 1973.)

Note: Dr. Rinse recommends that the amount of lecithin be *doubled* in severe cases of atherosclerosis (clogged arteries).

There is now some evidence to indicate that yogurt helps lower blood cholesterol, although this was not discovered until *after* Dr. Rinse formulated his supplement.

Step 4: Kick Your Bad Habits

When you indulge in bad habits and do not eat properly, it's absolutely essential to supplement your diet with selected nutrients if you want to protect your heart. But this does not mean that the use of supplements can justify a bad habit or a bad diet. If you really want to protect your heart and live longer than the average person, you should quit smoking cigarettes and stop eating junk foods. You should go easy on the use of coffee, alcohol, sugar, and salt. You should try to quit eating processed or convenience foods that may be loaded with sugar, fat, salt, refined carbohydrate, or artificial additives.

Film star *Terry Moore,* who wrote of her long association with ill-fated *Howard Hughes,* has remained healthy and beautiful by being independent and original in her health habits. It's important to use *informed* judgment in caring for your body if you want exceptional health.

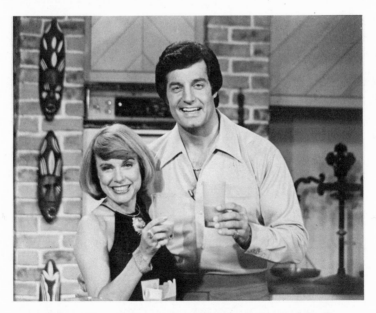

Actress Terry Moore, author of the book "Howard Be Thy Name," stays beautiful by following a health-care program that includes exercise as well as good nutrition.

It's absolutely imperative that you eat a balanced diet of fresh, natural foods to get all the nutrients you need for a healthy heart. Even if you supplemented your diet with every nutrient known to man, you'd still have to eat natural foods to get all the known and unknown nutrients you must have for good health. So it's just as important to eat properly as it is to kick your bad habits. *If you want to live longer than the average person and die of old age rather than from disease, you should not eat and live the way the average person does.* Don't hesitate to be different. Kick those bad habits now, even if everyone else refuses to do so.

Step 5: Reduce the Stress in Your Life

There are many theories about the cause of heart disease. According to *Dr. Meyer Friedman* and *Dr. Ray H. Rosenman,* authors of *Type A Behavior and Your Heart* (Alfred A. Knopf, Inc., 1974), the primary cause of heart disease is a distinct behavior pattern they call Type A Behavior. "In the absence of Type A Behavior Pattern," they maintain, "coronary heart disease almost never occurs before seventy years of age, regardless of the fatty foods eaten, the cigarettes smoked, or the lack of exercise. But when this behavior pattern *is* present, coronary heart disease can easily erupt in one's thirties or forties."

What is Type A Behavior? According to Friedman and Rosenman, it is a personality trait in which the individual is excessively competitive, aggressive, and impatient and has a harrying sense of time urgency. The individual simply runs himself to death trying to do too much in a short period of time.

There is no doubt that stress plays a role in the development of heart disease. But according to the authors of *Live Longer Now* (Grosset and Dunlap, 1974), "All the evidence seems to show that stress is, at best, only a minor factor in the cause of heart disease."

Regardless of what you hear about all the causes of heart disease, it makes good sense to do all you can to reduce or eliminate *all* the harmful influences in your life, including excessive stress. Remember, however, that what is stress for one person may be fun for another. A guest on a television talk show, for example, may undergo much more stress than the host who enjoys doing his show. An impatient truck driver fighting traffic and time schedules may experience more stress than a relaxed company president who takes time out to play golf occasionally. *Mental attitude* has a lot to do with whether stress is harmful or not.

Don't suppress your ambitions just to avoid stress. Everyday living is a form of stress. When you meet the challenges of life and accomplish something worthwhile, the satisfaction you experience may actually *contribute* to your longevity. Be guided by the way you feel and do what seems to make you happy. If you like to work, just make sure that you don't set your goals too high prematurely. Make your way one step at a time. Give yourself plenty of time to accomplish what you want to do in each step. Then, if you succeed, you can take the next step. Try to do what you *enjoy* doing. If you enjoy your work, you can be happy with a heavy workload. Your work can even be healthful if you get adequate rest and don't fight the clock.

WHAT YOU CAN DO TO
PREVENT CANCER IN YOUR BODY

Cancer, *the second most common cause of death,* is the most dreaded of all diseases. Few diseases destroy the body so completely before death as cancer does. Like a great parasite sucking the life blood of its victims, a cancerous growth drains the body until muscles and organs literally waste away from starvation. Detected early enough, some forms of cancer can be cut out of the body or be suppressed with chemical therapy or radiation. But the only guaranteed treatment for cancer is *prevention.* Fortunately, there is plenty that you can do to prevent many types of cancer.

If you smoke, you can greatly reduce your chances of developing lung and bladder cancer (as well as heart disease) simply by giving up smoking. Drinking alcohol increases susceptibility to cancer, especially when alcohol and cigarettes are combined. Refined and processed foods containing such additives as sodium nitrite are believed to cause cancer. Lack of adequate fiber in the diet slows bowel function so that unfriendly colon bacteria have plenty of time to convert bile acids to carcinogenic toxins. Excessive use of sugar contributes to the growth of unfriendly bacteria.

Whenever you have a choice, eat fresh, natural foods that are rich in bran and cellulose. Many celebrities add a couple teaspoons of miller's bran to each meal to make sure that they have adequate fiber for effective elimination and a healthy colon.

Cutting down the amount of fat in your diet will also help protect against cancer. This means cutting down on *all types* of fat—animal and vegetable. Don't increase your consumption of vegetable oil with the idea that more oil will prevent heart disease—it won't and it might cause cancer. If you cut down on your animal fat adequately, you won't need to add more than one or two tablespoons of vegetable oil to your diet. (Be sure to study the general dietary advice offered in Chapter 4.)

When there is any question at all about the effect that artificial sweeteners, food dyes, and other non-food items might have on your body, avoid them. Even if no one can prove that they cause cancer in humans, the fact that they can cause cancer in animals is reason enough to omit them from your diet. You don't need them. Anything that causes cancer in humans causes cancer in animals. So it's logical to assume that this works in reverse.

If you really want to protect your health, you shouldn't eat or drink anything that your body cannot use or does not need.

Nutritional Deficiencies Can Cause Cancer!

According to the U.S. Department of Agriculture (*Human Nutrition,* 1971), "The major known causes of cancer are felt to be viruses and cancer-producing chemicals in food and the environment . ... There is a small but growing body of data suggesting that chronic low-level of some nutrients is a factor in the incidence of cancer in man." So what you eat *can* be important in the prevention of cancer!

Recent research indicates that large doses of Vitamin A or Vitamin C might be effective in preventing the development of chemically induced cancer. We've all read recent news releases stating that Vitamin C taken with foods containing sodium nitrite prevents the chemical reaction that forms cancer-causing nitrosamines in the stomach. A few researchers are now experimenting with large doses of Vitamin A, Vitamin C, and other nutrients in the treatment of cancer with encouraging results. Research by the National Cancer Institute, for example, has shown that Vitamin C stimulates the body's defense mechanism to help prevent the spread of cancer in a diseased body. Vitamin C also strengthens the collagen that binds tissue cells together for greater resistance against invasion by cancer cells—as does Vitamin A. Antioxidant nutrients such as Vitamin E and selenium provide additional resistance by protecting cell membranes.

Obviously, it's not such a kooky idea for a healthy person to supplement a questionable diet with vitamins and minerals to *prevent* disease. And when disease does develop, it makes good sense to use large doses of vitamins as part of the treatment.

Cancer's Seven Danger Signals

A cancer victim is often unaware that he has the disease until it is detected in a routine medical examination. Very often, however, a medical examination will fail to reveal an existing malignancy. So even if you have a regular medical checkup, see your doctor immediately if you develop any unusual symptoms that last for two weeks or longer.

Here are cancer's seven danger signals:

1. Unusual bleeding or discharge. Bleeding from the rectum may only mean hemorrhoids, but it may also point to colon cancer, especially when there is a change in bowel habits. Vaginal bleeding after menopause always warrants a careful pelvic examination for uterine cancer, even if a Pap smear for cervical cancer is negative.

2. A lump or thickening in the breast or elsewhere. Most breast cancers are discovered by self examination. If you are a woman, you should examine your breasts regularly so that you can detect any sudden appearance or enlargement of a lump. Even if there are no lumps, watch for any type of discharge from your nipples. (Men should examine their testicles for lumps.)

3. A sore that does not heal. A sore anywhere on the body—on the skin or in the mouth—that fails to heal could develop into a malignancy. Pigmentation, lumps, or chronic bleeding on the skin should be examined for skin cancer. Unusual white or red spots in the mouth should be brought to the attention of a physician.

4. A change in bowel or bladder habits. A tumor or growth in the bowel can obstruct elimination or result in chronic diarrhea. Prostate cancer can block the flow of urine from the bladder (in men), while bladder or kidney cancer could result in blood in the urine.

5. Hoarseness or cough. Persistent hoarseness always calls for an examination of the larynx or voice box. Cancer of the vocal cords, for example, can cause hoarseness. Trouble anywhere in the throat, bronchial tubes, or lungs may result in a cough.

6. Indigestion or difficulty in swallowing. These symptoms may point to a malignancy in the throat, esophagus, or stomach. Bleeding from these areas will show up in the stool as a black discoloration resembling coffee grounds. Blood from the colon or rectal area will remain red.

7. Change in a wart or mole. Malignant melanoma, one of the most dangerous forms of cancer, may develop when a mole or birthmark begins to grow and blacken or if it ulcerates or bleeds. Any progressive change in a wart or mole should be a cause for concern.

Don't Ignore Any Unusual Symptoms

Any persistent ache or pain of unknown origin should be brought to the attention of a physician. An intractable backache, for example, that is not aggravated by movement or relieved by rest may have an internal origin, which could mean cancer. Backache caused by a tumor is usually felt 24 hours a day and is often worse at night—and it grows worse from week to week. Prostate cancer in men (usually after the age of 60), like bone cancer, can result in constant backache.

Chronic fatigue, enlarged lymph nodes, a tendency to bruise easily, and weight loss may point to possible "blood cancer," such as Hodgkin's disease or leukemia.

Don't ever delay seeing a doctor because of a fear of bad news. The sooner cancer is discovered the better your chances of being cured. A diagnosis of cancer is not an automatic death sentence. Many people, including such celebrities as *Van Johnson, Shirley Temple Black, Beverly Sills,* and *Arthur Godfrey,* have overcome cancer. You can, too, if you combine self help with professional care.

Actress *Amanda Blake* of "Gunsmoke" fame was cured of cancer that developed on the floor of her mouth after years of smoking two packs of cigarettes a day. It took her four months, however, to overcome her fear of treatment of cancer. "Fear is the killer," she warns. "Being afraid to get medical help—that's what kills you. So go to the doctor. Cancer is being cured every day."

Recommended reading: *Cancer: How to Prevent It and How to Help Your Doctor Fight It,* by George Berkley, Ph.D., Prentice-Hall, Inc., 1978.

HOW TO MAINTAIN GOOD BOWEL HEALTH

It is now well known that colon and rectum cancer can result from stagnation in the lower bowel. This is one reason you should do everything you can to avoid constipation. A clogged, overloaded colon in itself is uncomfortable and can result in headache, varicose veins, anal fissures, and other problems. So even if constipation is classified as a minor disorder, it can have serious consequences if it continues unrelieved.

Everyone suffers from constipation occasionally. Unaccustomed excitement, emotional stress, or a change in routine may temporarily "short circuit" the bowels. When that happens to you, don't panic and take a laxative. Chances are your bowels will resume their normal function in a day or two if you eat properly and visit the toilet regularly.

When you take a laxative, the artificial stimulation of the laxative may empty your small intestines as well as your large intestines. It may then be three or four days before you'll feel the urge to visit the toilet again. If you falsely assume that you're still constipated and take another laxative, you'll again prematurely empty your intestines. Repeated use of laxatives, either because of chronic constipation or laxative hangover, soon results in a dependency upon the use of laxatives. Your lower bowel may then refuse to function at all without the artificial stimulation of a commercial laxative.

Don't use laxatives. If you're already using them, gradually discontinue their use. You can restore normal bowel function by following our basic rules of bowel care.

Five Basic Rules of Bowel Care

**1. Visit the toilet at the same time each day, preferably after

breakfast. Once your bowels have been trained to empty at a certain time, nerve reflexes will trigger the expected urge.

2. Don't ever ignore an urge to empty your bowels, no matter when it occurs. Failure to empty a full colon may result in distension of the bowel, requiring a larger amount of waste matter in the colon to produce an urge for evacuation. Furthermore, when emptying of the colon is delayed, water is absorbed from the waste, leaving it hard and impacted.

3. Include plenty of raw fruits and vegetables in your diet. This will keep your colon supplied with the cellulose it needs to hold moisture and stimulate the growth of friendly bacteria.

4. Add a couple teaspoons of unprocessed miller's bran to each meal to make sure that you supply your intestines with enough fiber to stimulate bowel function.

5. Drink plenty of water during the day to keep the fiber in your bowels moist.

Will these basic rules work for the average person? Pricilla B. thinks so. "I suffered from chronic constipation for several years before I tried your basic rules," she told us in confidence. "Now, for the first time since I graduated from college, I don't have to take a laxative to go to the bathroom! My bowel habits are now a pleasure, and I feel so much better I can't believe it."

Note: While it's generally best to empty the bowels at least once a day, it's normal for some people to visit the toilet once every two or three days. If your stools are moist and well-formed, you're not constipated, no matter how infrequently you visit the toilet. If your bowels fail to move as usual, however, and your stool becomes hard and small, you may assume that you are constipated. You may then use an enema, when necessary, to empty your colon until your regularity is restored. (Fleet disposable enemas are handy when you are traveling.)

HOW TO FIGHT COLDS AND
INFECTIONS WITH VITAMIN C

Colds are not usually serious, but they are common. When they occur in a poorly resistant body they can lead to more serious infections, such as pneumonia, sinusitis, or bronchitis. A cold infection itself can lower the body's resistance to disease. Unfortunately, most people who are susceptible to colds experience recurring infections regularly with seasonal changes.

There is now considerable evidence to indicate that taking extra Vitamin C can increase resistance to colds as well as speed recovery from infection. It was discovered recently, for example, that large doses of Vitamin C stimulate the production of a protein substance in the body called *interferon,* which helps protect against disease and infection. A few doctors are now treating patients experimentally with interferon, but it is not yet available to the public. You can help your body produce its own interferon by taking Vitamin C. In addition to helping you combat cold infection, interferon will boost your body's defense system against many other diseases, including cancer.

How Much Vitamin C Do You Need?

The Food and Nutrition Board of the National Research Council maintains that 45 milligrams of Vitamin C daily is more than enough to maintain good health. But according to *Dr. Linus Pauling,* a biochemist who was awarded the Nobel Prize for chemistry in 1954, the amount of vitamin C needed for the best of health may range from 250 to 10,000 milligrams a day with an optimum rate of 1,000 to 2,000 milligrams a day for the average person. Dr. Pauling supplements his diet with 6,000 milligrams of Vitamin C daily.

Dr. Irwin Stone, a biochemist who wrote *The Healing Factor, Vitamin C Against Disease* after doing research on Vitamin C, takes from 10,000 to 20,000 milligrams of Vitamin C daily, which he mixes in liquids and sprinkles on food. It was Dr. Stone who first pointed out that man and other primates are unable to synthesize ascorbic acid (Vitamin C) because of a genetic mutation, making it necessary for them to consume large amounts of this vitamin for the best of health. (The average "good diet" of man supplies about 100 milligrams of Vitamin C daily. A gorilla consumes more than 4,000 milligrams of Vitamin C daily by eating large quantities of fresh vegetation. The bodies of other animals *manufacture* the equivalent of thousands of milligrams of Vitamin C daily. The amount of Vitamin C manufactured by a cat or a dog per kilogram of weight, for example, would equal 10,000 milligrams a day in a man weighing 154 pounds.)

Dr. Albert Szent-Gyorgyi, the physician who won a Nobel Prize for his discovery of Vitamin C in 1928, reported that he now takes from 1,000 to 2,000 milligrams of Vitamin C daily to prevent the cold infections that plagued him in his younger years. Dr. Szent-Gyorgyi is now in his mid-eighties. (Dr. Pauling is about eighty.)

You obviously cannot afford to ignore the advice of such outstanding scientists as Pauling, Stone, and Szent-Gyorgyi. Until the average person dies of old age rather than from disease, we cannot assume that the nutrient level recommended for the maintenance of "normal health" is necessarily adequate for the *best* of health.

If you want to take a little extra Vitamin C, go right ahead. We recommend it to all of our celebrity friends who work hard and who cannot afford to get sick. Our good friend *Aniko Farrell,* a former "Miss Canada" and "Miss World" who now sings and acts, has learned from experience that Vitamin C helps protect her from colds. "When I'm doing a show," she told us, "I take plenty of Vitamin C to make sure that I don't catch a cold. And, believe me, it works! I cannot afford to get sick because there are no understudies in summer stock."

Actor *Joseph Campanella,* who is in great demand as an announcer, narrator, emcee, and commercial spokesman must make a special effort to avoid colds to protect his voice. "I can generally anticipate a cold," he says. "I can sense way back in my throat when I'm going to catch a cold. I'll use a good antiseptic gargle such as Listerine and maybe take *one* antihistamine. I also take some extra Vitamin C. I repeat this procedure the next day if I still have symptoms. I have one slight cold a year that may last a day or so and that's all."

Gwynne Gilford of "Waverly's Wonders" takes Vitamin C tablets to prevent colds. "But when I begin to feel the onslaught of a cold," she adds, "I take orange juice or grapefruit juice with honey along with Vitamin C."

You can determine for yourself how much Vitamin C is best for you. There are, however, some precautions to be observed when taking large doses of Vitamin C.

HOME TREATMENT WITH MEGA-C

Since Vitamin C is water soluble, any excess will be eliminated by your kidneys. You can reduce this loss by taking Vitamin C in divided doses. For example, if you want to take 1,500 milligrams daily, you can take 500 milligrams with each meal. This way, the vitamin will be available for use by your body throughout the day. Taking too large a dose at one time forces your body to eliminate what it cannot use immediately. If you take Vitamin C only once a day, and your body needs more of the vitamin than usual, there may not be adequate Vitamin C in your blood a few hours after taking the vitamin.

If you become ill and you want to keep your blood saturated with Vitamin C, try taking 500 milligrams or more of Vitamin C every two hours for a few days. Cut back on the dosage if you experience diarrhea. Take your largest doses after meals. Most people will experience diarrhea if they take 3,000 milligrams or more of Vitamin C on an empty stomach. Once you become accustomed to taking Vitamin C, you'll be less likely to experience diarrhea from large doses.

Persons suffering from gouty arthritis, kidney stones (formed from uric acid, cystine, or calcium oxalate), an inflamed bladder, or any other condition aggravated by an acid urine may have to be cautious about taking large doses of ascorbic acid (Vitamin C). Sodium ascorbate, a buffered form of Vitamin C, will not acidify the urine, but persons on a low-salt (low-sodium) diet must avoid consuming anything containing sodium additives, including sodium ascorbate. If you find it necessary to take ascorbate in combination with calcium, magnesium, zinc, or some other mineral, ask you doctor which will be best for you.

You should discontinue the use of any Vitamin C supplement the day before a scheduled urinalysis when testing the urine for sugar. Vitamin C is chemically similar to glucose and might result in a false reading when present in the urine.

Whenever you discontinue the use of large doses of Vitamin C following recovery from illness, it might be a good idea to reduce the dosage *gradually* over a period of a week or two until you revert to your usual dosage. This will prevent a possible rebound effect caused by a sudden decrease in the amount of Vitamin C in your blood. When the body is accustomed to receiving large doses of Vitamin C, some of the ascorbic acid in the blood is converted to other substances by enzymes. If Vitamin C is suddenly withdrawn, enzymatic activity may continue to remove Vitamin C from the blood, temporarily resulting in a lowered resistance to infection. Tapering off large doses of Vitamin C will give your body time to curtail its production of the enzymes used in the conversion of Vitamin C.

Recommended reading: *Vitamin C, the Common Cold, and the Flu,* by Dr. Linus Pauling, W.H. Freeman and Company, 1976.

SUPERNUTRITION AND MEGAVITAMIN THERAPY

With all the talk these days about supernutrition and mega-vitamin therapy, you might want to try taking large doses of vitamins for special effects or to speed recovery from illness. If you do, you should know enough about vitamins to use them effectively and to protect yourself against a possible overdose. Remember that what is best for one person may not be best for you. *Peter Lupus,* who was recently voted the "Best Built Actor of the Year," takes 150 protein-vitamin-mineral tablets each day to supplement a specially formulated diet. Actor *Ted Knight* also takes 150 pills a day, which he says keeps him in "great shape." *George Hamilton* supplements his diet with 120 pills daily—40 with each meal. It's not likely that you'll find it necessary to take so many pills. But that's for you to decide. Just remember that supplements are not a substitute for food. You cannot possibly get all the fiber, nutrients, enzymes, and other elements your body needs from pills alone. Besides, there are many undiscovered nutrients in natural foods, and you need *all* of them for the best of health. So no matter how many vitamins you take, you should make a special effort to eat properly and then use vitamin pills as a dietary supplement.

Note: Diabetics, persons taking blood thinners, and pregnant women should not experiment with large doses of vitamins without a doctor's supervision.

Vitamin A and Low-Fat Diets

If you are on a low-fat diet, you may need to take a Vitamin A supplement. The carotene in green and yellow fruits and vegetables can be converted to Vitamin A in your body, but Vitamin A supplied by food is absorbed in the presence of fat. For this reason, low-fat diets tend to be deficient in Vitamin A.

The recommended daily allowance for Vitamin A is 5,000 units. There is evidence to indicate that some individuals may need as much as 25,000 units daily for the best of health. Since Vitamin A is fat soluble, it can be stored in your body. So you'd have to be cautious about taking large amounts of the vitamin over a period of several months. Anyone can safely take up to 20,000 units of Vitamin A daily. (A two-ounce serving of cooked beef liver provides more than 30,000 units of Vitamin A.) When there is a Vitamin A deficiency or a medical problem requiring therapeutic doses of Vitamin A, a doctor may prescribe up to 50,000 units a day for a few months.

Vitamin A is sometimes prescribed in the treatment of infections, skin conditions, and cancer. When you do take Vitamin A, be sure to take some additional Vitamin E.

Don't Separate the B Vitamins

There are several B vitamins—and they all work together. Taking only one B vitamin might result in a deficiency in other B vitamins. So if you're taking B vitamins for nutritional insurance, you should take them all together, in a B complex formula. Since B vitamins are water soluble, any excess will be eliminated by your kidneys. None of the B vitamins are stored in your body. You must have a fresh supply each day. Meats, liver, brewer's yeast, and wheat germ are good sources of all the B vitamins.

Vitamin B complex is most often prescribed for nervous and metabolic disorders. The most popular dosage is about 50 milligrams of each of the B vitamins. Reduce the dosage if heart palpitations or any other symptoms occur. Large doses of niacin (Vitamin B_3) may result in a temporary (and harmless) flushing or redness of the skin. (This reaction does not occur with niacinamide.)

Vitamin C: The Most
Useful Vitamin in Home Care

Vitamin C is believed to be useful in strengthening tissue cells, combating infection, delaying the aging process, neutralizing toxins, reducing blood cholesterol, preventing cancer, speeding healing, strengthening blood vessels, recharging the adrenal glands, and generally aiding the body in many other ways. Vitamin C is virtually nontoxic, so anyone can safely take several hundred milligrams a day. Since excess Vitamin C is eliminated by the kidneys, large doses will result in frequent urination. An overdose will result in diarrhea. There are a few precautions to be observed when taking very large doses of Vitamin C under special circumstances. Turn back and re-read the material under the heading "Home Treatment with Mega-C."

Note: Vitamin C facilitates absorption of iron and calcium. If you are anemic and you take iron, or if you need additional calcium in your bones, add Vitamin C to your supplements.

Delay Aging with Vitamin E

Most standard medical references maintain that Vitamin E in excess of the recommended daily allowance (RDA) of 15 international units offers no known benefits to the human body. There is an abundance of literature stating an opinion to the contrary, however. Since Vitamin E is believed to be a natural anticoagulant, for example, many doctors recommend daily divided doses of several hundred units or more to relieve or prevent the formation of blood clots in special cases. *Dr. Alton Ochsner* of the Ochsner Clinic in New Orleans states emphatically that large doses of the alpha tocopheryl component of Vitamin E materially reduce the incidence of venous thrombosis and pulmonary embolism in surgical patients. "After a 25-year experience with the use of alpha tocopheryl, both immediately after the operation in the severely ill patient and in the longterm use of it in patients who have a tendency toward thrombosis, I am convinced that it is of real value," he reported in a 1976 edition of *Executive Health* (No. 5, Rancho Santa Fe, California).

Vitamin E is also an antioxidant, and in recent years has been labeled an anti-aging nutrient. It's now well known that Vitamin E protects tissue cells and essential fatty acids from the destructive effects of oxygen. Many people who do not eat adequate amounts of resh vegetables and whole-grain products do not even take in the 15 units daily needed for minimum protection.

Like Vitamin A, Vitamin E is a fat-soluble vitamin, but there is no evidence to date to indicate that fairly large doses of Vitamin E are harmful. Most celebrities who take Vitamin E to combat the aging process take from 200 to 400 units daily.

If you want to try taking large doses of Vitamin E, begin with 100 units a day and slowly increase the dosage over a period of several weeks if no adverse effects occur. (Doctors use up to 300 units a day in correcting deficiencies.)

Note: When taking Vitamin E for general health purposes, it might be best to take *mixed* tocopherols, which contain all the components of Vitamin E as found in nature. You may take Vitamin E with meals, but don't take it with iron supplements.

Recommended reading: *Supernutrition,* by Richard Passwater, Ph.D., Dial Press, 1975.

SUMMARY

1. Six of the ten leading causes of death, including heart disease and cancer, can often be *prevented* with proper attention to diet!

2. Most people can benefit from general use of dietary supplements, but remember that supplements should not be substituted for fresh, natural foods in a balanced diet.

3. Supplements containing Vitamins C and E are popular because they offer such a wide range of benefits in preventing disease and delaying the aging process.

4. You should not eat and live the way the average person does if you want to die of old age rather than from disease.

5. Your chances of preventing cancer, heart disease, and other killers are better if you give up such bad habits as smoking cigarettes and drinking alcohol and then make a special effort to avoid refined and processed foods.

6. Eating fresh fruits and vegetables and adding unprocessed miller's bran to your diet will help prevent constipation and colon cancer.

7. Large amounts of Vitamin C taken in daily divided doses may help protect against infection and disease (from colds to cancer) by stimulating the production of interferon in your body.

8. When taking large doses of vitamins in a megavitamin program, there are precautions to be observed and certain limitations that should not be exceeded without a doctor's supervision.

9. Anyone who is not pregnant, diabetic, or taking blood thinners can safely take 1,000 milligrams of Vitamin C, 200 units of Vitamin E, and 10,000 units of Vitamin A along with a moderately potent Vitamin B complex in daily divided doses.

10. Always heed the warning signals of your body and see your doctor when you experience persistent symptoms of any kind.

9

How Hard-Working Celebrities Fight Fatigue and Depression To Stay Mentally Alert

Chronic fatigue is a common complaint among Americans. So is depression. About one out of every seven Americans can expect to suffer from severe clinical depression at least once during a lifetime.

There are many mental and physical causes of fatigue and depression. Most diseases result in fatigue, which, if unrelieved, can lead to depression. *Chronic fatigue may be the first warning you have that something is wrong with your body.* Always seek the help of a physician in translating fatigue and other symptoms into a diagnosis.

Fortunately, most of the common causes of fatigue are not serious and can be corrected with such simple measures as rest, diet, and mind control. Some types of fatigue, such as that experienced by persons who sit all day, can be relieved by exercising. Different types of fatigue require different measures. There are, however, some basic procedures that *everyone* should follow to prevent or relieve the common causes of fatigue. A good diet, for example, can be recommended for anyone. Food supplements can be used to offset the stresses, deficiencies, and contaminants that are part of our modern way of life. Tension-relieving procedures that relax muscles and assure adequate sleep can be used beneficially by everyone. Tips on how to recognize and control emotional stress may help prevent heart attacks as well as conserve energy. All of this will help prevent the agonizing depression that occurs when mental and physical stress combine to break the human spirit.

YOU CAN BENEFIT FROM THE EXPERIENCE OF CELEBRITIES

Celebrities are constantly fighting fatigue and depression. A movie or television actor who is working has a long and fatiguing day. Meals are often irregular and nutritionally inadequate. Nervous strain makes it difficult to sleep at night. Even if an actor has a job, it's often temporary, resulting in a great deal of anxiety and insecurity about the future. An actor who is unemployed must worry about today as well as tomorrow.

Actors are subjected to practically all of the common causes of fatigue. Yet, they must stay well enough to accept a new assignment on a moment's notice. They must always be mentally alert to learn new lines and follow cues.

We can all learn from actors and celebrities who must daily fight fatigue and depression to survive. Many of the suggestions outlined in this chapter have been gleaned from the advice and activities of our celebrity friends who are healthy as well as successful. What they do to fight fatigue and depression can be included in your own body-improvement program.

WHAT TO DO ABOUT HYPOGLYCEMIA, A COMMON CAUSE OF FATIGUE

Once considered to be a rare condition, hypoglycemia (low blood sugar) is becoming increasingly more common in America. Brain cells as well as muscle fibers feed upon blood sugar. When blood sugar falls below a certain level, symptoms may range from inability to think clearly to agonizing fatigue.

Rarely, hypoglycemia can be caused by a pancreatic tumor or some other organic disorder. In the *organic* type of hypoglycemia, the fasting blood sugar level is consistently low, resulting in chronic fatigue. In *functional* hypoglycemia, the most common form of low blood sugar, the fasting blood sugar may be normal. But eating or drinking something containing sugar or refined carbohydrate produces a surge of energy that is followed by a sudden *drop* in blood sugar a few hours later. This results in unbearable fatigue and a craving for sweets. If sugar or some other refined carbohydrate is consumed, however, a surge of energy will again be followed by a drop in blood sugar a few hours later. A vicious cycle develops in which the victim of hypoglycemia is constantly snacking to relieve fatigue and hunger, resulting in an addiction to refined carbohydrates.

Jarvis R., a bus driver, was a victim of functional hypoglycemia. Often, when he was driving his bus on a long trip, he developed a headache that was accompanied by weakness, trembling, and inability to think clearly. "The only thing that seems to help me is a snack," Jarvis observed. "But the lift doesn't last long, so I have to keep snacking. If I don't have any candy in my pocket, I have to stop the bus somewhere and pick up something at a store." Once, when Jarvis was carrying a full load of passengers, he had a near-disastrous accident. "I just couldn't think clearly," he complained. "I couldn't act quickly enough when I saw the accident coming." Fortunately, no one was seriously hurt. When Jarvis told us about the accident, we told him how he might be able to prevent future accidents by keeping his blood sugar under control—by eating to prevent hypoglycemia. The results were immediate. When we saw Jarvis a week later, he told us that he felt better the same day he started our diet. "I haven't had a headache all week long," he reported gratefully, "and I feel stronger and more alert. If I have another accident, it won't be my fault!"

If you drive a car, or fly a plane, you, too, should know how to prevent hypoglycemia to protect yourself and others.

How You Can Prevent Hypoglycemia

Carbohydrate is the best and cleanest source of energy for the human body. But the carbohydrate should come from fresh, *natural* foods and not from refined or processed foods. When you eat sugar, white flour, refined cereals, and other forms of refined carbohydrates, they are absorbed so rapidly that your blood sugar is suddenly greatly elevated. Your pancreas must then secrete a large amount of insulin to remove the excess blood sugar for storage. After years of eating refined carbohydrates, your pancreas may become so sensitive that it shoots an excessive amount of insulin into your blood at the slightest provocation. The result is that every time you eat something containing sugar or white flour, a sudden elevation in blood sugar triggers a pancreatic reaction. A flood of insulin then removes an excessive amount of sugar from your blood, causing weakness, fatigue, hunger, and other symptoms. A desire to eat or drink something sweet may be irresistible.

Obviously, frequent snacking prompted by a fluctuating blood sugar level can lead to obesity and other physical problems. Your pancreas may eventually become exhausted, resulting in diabetes.

The caffeine in coffee and colas (even when sugar-free) can contribute to the development of hypoglycemia and diabetes by stimulating the adrenal glands (which trigger the release of stored sugar into the blood). A sensitive pancreas will react to this sudden elevation of blood sugar just as it does when sugar is eaten. Forcing your body to store blood sugar as glycogen by eating excessive amounts of sugar and other refined carbohydrates and then triggering the release of glycogen as sugar by drinking coffee and colas all day is bound to speed the development of diabetes.

Since Americans eat huge amounts of refined carbohydrates and drink huge amounts of coffee and colas (see Chapter 4), it's no wonder that both hypoglycemia and diabetes are so common in America. *The obvious solution to this problem is to quit eating sugar, white-flour products, and refined cereals and to cut down on the consumption of coffee and colas.* Your body can get all the carbohydrate it needs from such natural carbohydrates as fruits, vegetables, and whole-grain products. The complex carbohydrate supplied by natural foods is absorbed slowly and won't overstimulate your pancreas with sudden elevations in blood sugar.

Should You Undergo a
Glucose Tolerance Test?

A diagnosis of functional hypoglycemia is usually made according to the results of a five-hour glucose tolerance test. Blood sugar is tested at intervals over a five-hour period after the subject drinks a solution sweetened with glucose. If the pancreas overreacts, there will be an abnormal drop in blood sugar a few hours after the test begins, accompanied by weakness, trembling, sweating, hunger, and other symptoms of hypoglycemia.

If you suspect that you are suffering from functional hypoglycemia, you may do one of two things: (1) You can ask your doctor for a glucose tolerance test, or (2) you may go ahead and make the recommended changes in your diet. A glucose tolerance test is a brutal procedure in which blood must be drawn from the arm several times. Most of us would not be anxious to undergo such a test. Besides, the test is often difficult to interpret, and *symptoms* may be more meaningful than the results of the test. For example, a diagnosis of hypoglycemia is not usually made unless blood sugar falls below 40 milligrams per 100 milliliters of blood. Yet, some persons may experience symptoms at higher levels if readings drop sharply. So, if you have any of the symptoms of hypoglycemia, you should make the recommended changes in your diet even if the test results are negative according to medical standards.

Actually, the type of diet used to prevent or relieve the symptoms of functional hypoglycemia is the type of diet we should all follow anyway. Simple dietary measures will relieve the symptoms of functional hypoglycemia, making it unnecessary to undergo a glucose tolerance test. If symptoms persist in spite of following the recommended diet, you should have a complete medical checkup in case you have an organic problem.

A Diet to Relieve
the Symptoms of Hypoglycemia

The first thing you should do to get your blood sugar under control is to *eliminate sugar, white-flour products, refined cereals, and other refined carbohydrates from your diet.* In addition to overloading your pancreas, such foods are deficient in the chromium, B vitamins, and other nutrients your body needs to metabolize carbohydrate. Refined foods will, in fact, create a deficiency in essential nutrients.

Eat a variety of fresh, natural foods. Select whole-grain breads and cereals. Avoid processed foods. Do not use sweeteners of any kind except fresh and dried fruits. Remember that canned and bottled foods often contain refined sugar. So be sure to stick to *fresh* foods.

Snack on protein-rich foods between meals. Keep cottage cheese or plain yogurt (with fresh fruit if desired), baked chicken, boiled eggs, skimmed milk, or toasted soybeans handy for a light snack between meals. Slow absorption of the protein supplied by these foods will provide you with energy as well as keep your blood sugar up. If you're not overweight, you can snack on peanut butter (with whole-grain wafers), raw nuts, Cheddar cheese, and other high calorie but protein-rich foods. (Don't eat processed cheese! And get your peanut butter from a health food store.)

If you snack on strictly natural foods between meals, chances are you'll eat less at mealtime. Best of all, you won't experience the midmorning, midafternoon, and midnight fatigue and hunger that generate a craving for sweets.

That's all there is to it! Following such simple guidelines can eliminate a variety of symptoms and forego the need for expensive medical tests. We recommend these guidelines to all of our celebrity friends who complain of fatigue. Those who are suffering from functional hypoglycemia always report relief from symptoms within a few days.

Since most doctors consider hypoglycemia to be a rare condition, it's often overlooked, even when symptoms are severe. *Burt Reynolds,* of "Smokey and the Bandit" fame, for example, suffered from a "mysterious illness" for many months before doctors finally discovered that he was a victim of hypoglycemia. "I was sick for a whole year," he stated in recalling his ordeal. "At the beginning nobody could figure out what was wrong with me. I was so sick I honestly thought I'd die."

Today, Burt Reynolds keeps his blood sugar under control by following a diet very similar to the one we outlined earlier in this chapter. "Hypoglycemia is something I'm going to have to live with the rest of my life," Burt says, "but at least it is now under control."

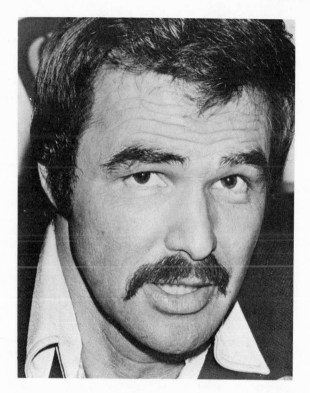

*Actor Burt Reynolds keeps his energy level up and
controls a blood sugar problem by following a special diet
that excludes sugar and refined carbohydrates.*

DIETARY SUPPLEMENTS
TO COMBAT FATIGUE

If you take supplements to increase your energy, be sure to include Vitamin B complex. Your body uses B vitamins in converting carbohydrates into energy. The more refined carbohydrates you eat the more B vitamins you need. *Brewer's yeast combined with desiccated liver* supplies all the B vitamins, plus the chromium and other nutrients you body needs to control blood sugar. Brewer's yeast is commonly used in energy drinks (see Chapter 10).

Wheat germ oil contains a substance called octacosanol that is believed to be an antifatigue factor. (If you have a health-drink formula that calls for vegetable oil, try using wheat germ oil.) Liver also contains an antifatigue factor. This is one reason why desiccated live is often combined with brewer's yeast in supplements.

Antioxidant nutrients such as Vitamin C, Vitamin E, pangamate (Vitamin B$_{15}$), and selenium might help combat fatigue by improving the body's use of oxygen. When *Muhammad Ali* regained the world heavyweight boxing crown for a record-breaking third time, he attributed his stamina and endurance to vitamins prescribed by comedian *Dick Gregory.* Orange juice laced with Vitamin E, magnesium, and bee pollen may have provided oxygen-conserving nutrients.

Beware of Low-Calorie Diets

Whatever type of diet you follow, remember that a diet that is too low in calories, even if it consists of natural foods, can result in nutritional deficiencies and fatigue. According to *Dr. E. Cheraskin,* the author of *Psychodietetics* (Stein and Day, 1974), a diet that supplies fewer than 2,100 to 2,400 calories daily can deprive you of vitamins and minerals that are essential for good health.

Presently, there are about 45 nutrients that are known to be vital in human nutrition. It seems likely, however, that many more essential nutrients will be discovered in natural foods. Since all of these nutrients cannot be supplied by supplements, it's not a good idea to stay on a low-calorie diet for very long, no matter how many supplements you take. It would be better to cut calories only moderately and then exercise so that you can continue to eat generous amounts of a variety of natural foods. This way, you can be assured of getting all the nutrients you need to be healthy and energetic. Also, muscles strengthened by exercise will help combat fatigue by providing you with enough reserve strength to get you through each day with strength to spare. So be sure to exercise, even if you take supplements.

HOW TO COPE WITH STRESS
AND NERVOUS TENSION

Unrelieved tension is a common cause of fatigue. When muscles are tight and tense because of emotional distress, energy stores are depleted and nerves are frayed. Fatigue caused by exercise can be beneficial, but chronic fatigue resulting from unrelieved nervous tension is exhausting and harmful.

According to Dr. Hans Selye, the author of *The Stress of Life* (McGraw-Hill, 1956), high blood pressure, gastric and duodenal ulcers, many nervous and emotional disturbances, and certain types of rheumatic, allergic, and cardiovascular and renal diseases can be caused by the tension of unrelieved stress. So can headache, colitis, skin disorders, and a host of other disorders. You know from reading Chapter 8 that the tension resulting from Type A Behavior is a common cause of heart disease. For the sake of your heart, don't let nervous tension get out of control. A certain amount of stress and tension is normal and harmless. When it grips your body 24 hours a day, however, excited nerves and a flood of adrenalin will literally burn you out. Worst of all, fatigue resulting from unrelieved stress and tension will make you more susceptible to almost any disease, even cancer.

You Can Control Your Mind and Body

Since most nervous tension originates in the mind, it can be controlled by the mind. With a little mental effort, you can literally erase worry from your mind and *command* your muscles to relax. With the right mental attitude, you can live with failure, disappointment, and adversity. You can be happy with what you have and who you are. This does not mean that you should not make an effort to forge ahead in improving your position in life. It means that you should be realistic in your goals and that you should be satisfied with your best effort, whatever the results. As Dr. Selye puts it, "Fight always for the highest attainable aim, but never put up resistance in vain."

When you have done the best you can, end the day by erasing the blackboard in your mind. Mentally flip the switches that redirect your thoughts. It might be necessary to exercise or participate in some form of recreational activity in order to clear your mind. Remember that if you go to bed each night with nervous tension caused by a cluttered mind, inability to sleep may lead to the type of fatigue that contributes to the development of depression.

How Celebrities Combat Stress
and Tension to Prevent Depression

Doris Day uses will power to combat depression. "Barring our depressed reactions to the few actual tragedies in our lives, the sensation of 'feeling low' seldom has anything to do with reality," she explains. "So I simply *refuse* to allow such sensations to take hold of me."

Gavin MacLeod also uses mind power to prevent depression. "I don't get myself mentally depressed," he states emphatically. "I talk to myself." *Olivia Newton-John* talks to her dogs!

When *Polly Bergen* feels low, she locks herself away from everyone and reads a book or listens to music. "Most importantly," she adds, "I try to control my feelings before they get control of me."

When depression does develop, exercise is often effective in providing a lift. "I play tennis," says *Charlton Heston.* "Expending physical energy is a great means of improving your state of mind." In addition to tennis, Heston runs two miles every morning for exercise. *Clint Eastwood* jogs or works out at home.

Helen Reddy also plays tennis. "I go out on the tennis court and bang hell out of the ball!" she exclaims.

If you don't enjoy exercising, there are many things you can do to change your state of mind. *George Kennedy* goes flying. *Lee Marvin* fishes. *Barbara Feldon* goes to lunch with a friend. *Dody Goodman* goes shopping, or she calls a friend to chat. "One sure way to forget all about yourself," she advises, "is to get involved with someone else."

Michael Landon does needlepoint or works a crossword puzzle. "Something that doesn't take too much concentrated effort," he suggests. "Just enough to get your mind off what was troubling you in the first place." *Henry Fonda* also does needlepoint—or he works in his garden.

Angie Dickinson puts her own problems into perspective by observing the problems of others. "Occasionally," she says, "I'll read the front page of the newspaper to get a sense of everybody else's problems. Then mine seem relatively insignificant."

If nothing else works, go ahead and cry! Psychologist *Dr. Joyce Brothers* says that "When I'm sad, I just give in and cry . . . . Then, after I've had my fill of crying, I take a swim. Exercise is definitely the best way to get over an upset."

A Muscle Control Routine
for Relieving Tension

One simple and popular method of relieving nervous tension is to employ procedures that relax the muscles. It's well known that depression and nervous tension are expressed in muscular tension. When the muscles are totally relaxed, nerves are also relaxed and the mind is relieved.

Many people are not aware that they have tense muscles. They walk around with clenched fists, contracted neck muscles, and a furrowed brow—and many of them *sleep* that way! If you are a chronically tense person, you probably cannot distinguish between a relaxed muscle and a tense muscle. You may have to *train* your muscles to relax.

How to relax: Lie in bed or on a carpeted floor so that you'll be comfortable. Begin with the muscles of your forehead. Wrinkle your brow as tightly as possible (with vertical furrows); then let the muscles of your face sag. Contract and relax your brow several times until you are sure that your facial muscles are relaxed.

Try to keep your facial muscles relaxed while you systematically contract and relax the other muscles of your body, going from one muscle to another. Concentrate on letting your muscles sag until you are as limp as a dishrag.

After you have practiced contracting and relaxing your muscles for a few weeks, you'll be able to distinguish tense muscles from relaxed muscles. In fact, chances are you'll be able to relax your muscles at will. Remember that if you can keep the muscles of your forehead relaxed it's not likely that the other muscles of your body will get too tense.

Cindy Williams and *Penny Marshall* practice a relaxing yoga routine on the set of "Laverne and Shirley" to relieve tension. "We usually end up with a relaxation exercise where we lie on the floor and relax every muscle in our body," says Cindy.

Note: Always take a little extra Vitamin C when you are under stress. It takes a considerable amount of Vitamin C for your adrenal glands to produce adrenalin. A Vitamin C deficiency created by adrenal activity can contribute greatly to the development of fatigue.

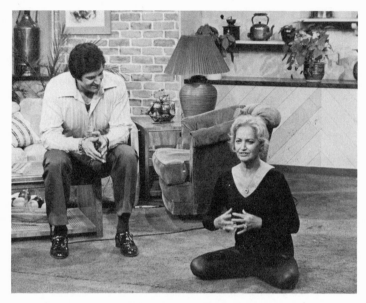

*Yoga master Rochelle Mark recommends yoga postures
to relieve tension and to prevent depression.*

Smoking cigarettes can also contribute to fatigue and tension. The nicotine absorbed from cigarette smoke in the mouth or in the lungs, in addition to stimulating nerves and constricting blood vessels, destroys Vitamin C in your blood. So if you really want to be relaxed and energetic, don't smoke!

HOW TO REJUVENATE
YOUR MIND AND BODY WITH SLEEP

A good night's sleep is the best medicine in the world for fatigue! When you sleep soundly, energy stores are replenished, waste products are disposed of, tissue cells and organs are repaired, your mind and body are refreshed, and your enthusiasm for living is restored.

Unfortunately, about 50 million Americans complain of sleep problems and about 25 million of these suffer from insomnia. Some of the reasons for sleep problems are obvious. Drinking coffee and tea with evening meals, for example, overeating before bedtime, lack of environmental control in sleeping quarters, worry caused by poor management of money, and so on, can make it impossible to sleep soundly every night.

When you lose too much sleep, you'll eventually fall asleep. Your body will always get the sleep it needs to survive. But inability to sleep soundly *every night* can have adverse effects on your performance during the day. And fatigue caused by lack of adequate sleep can make you more susceptible to disease and infection. You should, therefore, do all you can to make sure that nothing interferes with your sleep.

How Much Sleep Do You Need?

Most adults need from seven to nine hours of sleep each night. Some people seem to need only a small amount of sleep. The late *Lyndon B. Johnson*, for example, got by on four hours of sleep a night. If you sleep only four or five hours a night under conditions that are ideal for sleeping, and you don't feel sleepy during the day, you may be getting all the sleep you need. Just make sure that you give your body every opportunity to get all the sleep it needs, whether for five hours or for nine hours.

Lucille Ball says that she hasn't slept more than five hours a night for the past 25 years. "Several years ago," she explained, "I decided not to worry about the fact that I couldn't sleep. I get a lot of reading done. I work a lot of crossword puzzles. I get up and play cards, clean closets, or sew. Sometimes I'll go out into my garden in the middle of the night and take care of my plants . . . . Not sleeping doesn't bother me."

Lynda Day George told us that she didn't feel well when she slept too much. "I need only five or six hours of sleep a night," she said. "If I get more than that, I feel soggy all day."

Not everyone can get by on so little sleep. *Gavin MacLeod* for example, said that he functions best with eight hours of sleep. Obviously, we're all different, and we have different needs. Most of us, however, need around eight hours of sleep each night.

If you are consistently unable to sleep soundly at night and you feel tired and worn out during the day, there may be some medical reason why you cannot sleep. An overactive thyroid gland, for example, can keep your nerves on edge. Insomnia can be a symptom of depression or mèntal illness. Be sure to see your doctor if there is no obvious reason for your inability to sleep.

Except in the case of illness or a night job, it's rarely a good idea to sleep during the day. If you nap around the clock, you should not expect to sleep soundly at night. Don't get into the habit of sleeping during the day if you have trouble sleeping at night. And don't make the mistake of taking sleeping pills to *make* you sleep. You can count on your body to put you to sleep when the demand for sleep is great enough. There are many things you can do to help you sleep without taking drugs or medicine.

CELEBRITY TRICKS FOR CONQUERING INSOMNIA

Celebrities, like everyone else, often have trouble sleeping. Here are some of the tricks that a few of them employ to get a good night's sleep.

Brenda Vaccaro uses a muscle-relaxing routine similar to the one described earler in this chapter. "I just relax all over," she says. "First the toes, then the calves, then the knees, and so on all over my body."

Sandy Duncan achieves relaxation with self-hypnosis. "I talk first to my feet and slowly work my way up," she explained. "Usually it takes a few times through this routine to achieve total brain shutdown."

Dinah Shore goes for a midnight swim. *Olivia de Havilland* works crossword puzzles or reads something from the Bible. *Cary Grant* listens to classical music.

Carol Burnett uses a yoga routine. Here's what she recommends: "You lie in bed flat on your back with no pillow and inhale through your nose for four counts, then hold your breath for 16 counts, and finally exhale for eight counts . .... This kind of breathing slows down and regulates the heart beat. I usually go out very rapidly."

Danny Thomas simply takes a hot bath and drinks a glass of hot milk.

Kris Kristofferson offers this explanation for insomnia: "If you don't go to sleep, it's because you haven't worked hard enough, or played hard enough, or loved hard enough—but you can correct that."

John Davidson plays hard to aid sleeping. "I have to be physically tired," he says, "A good game of tennis or scuba diving knocks me out right away."

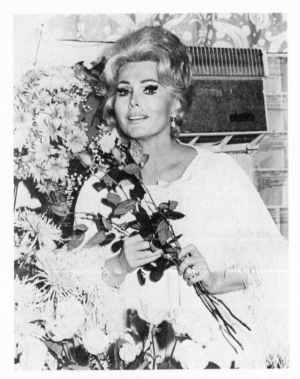

*TV personality Zsa Zsa Gabor, a former "Miss Hungary,"
says that sex is the best remedy for insomnia.*

Zsa Zsa Gabor recommends *sex* for insomnia. "I make love," she said in reply to a question about sleep remedies.

Phyllis Diller says that when she can't sleep, she calls Paul Newman to see if he is still married to Joanne Woodward. Then she cries herself to sleep.

Five Self-Help Procedures to Help You Sleep

Comedian *W. C. Fields* once said that "The best cure for insomnia is to get a lot of sleep." This is easier said than done. There are, however, certain basic procedures that *everyone* should follow in seeking a good night's sleep. No matter who you are, what you do, or what your problem is, you can benefit from the following procedures.

Procedure 1: Establish regular sleeping hours. Try to go to bed at the same time each night. Make sure that you allow yourself enough bed time to get adequate sleep. After you have spent several weeks on a regular sleeping schedule, you'll be able to determine exactly how much sleep you need.

Don't stay in bed unnecessarily. When you go to bed on time and wake up on time, get out of bed. Lying in bed for extra hours when you don't need to sleep slows the circulation of the blood and contributes to sluggishness that may persist for hours after you get out of bed. (Heart attacks and blood clots are more likely to occur when prolonged bed rest contributes to a slowdown in circulation.) Most of us find it necessary to spend one-third of our lives sleeping. But few of us can afford to waste precious hours by lying in bed unnecessarily. So don't go to bed except to rest, sleep, make love, or recover from illness.

Procedure 2: Avoid intense mental or physical activity late in the evening. Mild physical fatigue induced by moderate exercise helps promote sleep, but physical exhaustion will deter sleep. Don't wear yourself out in competitive physical activity late at night. And don't stimulate your brain with the intense concentration needed to perform an aggravating chore. Finish dreaded chores early in the afternoon so that you can relax and unwind in the evening. Spend the last few hours before bedtime doing something you *enjoy* doing.

Remember than an uncompleted job can monopolize your thoughts after you turn off the lights at night. Try to schedule your work so that you can end each day at a stopping point that will satisfy your sense of accomplishment as well as serve as a starting point for the next day.

Procedure 3: Don't overeat or drink coffee or tea in the evening. A light snack before bedtime helps promote sleep by drawing blood from the brain to the stomach. An overloaded stomach, however, may make it impossible to fall asleep soon after going to bed. *The first four hours of sleep are usually the soundest and therefore the most important.* If you have to toss and turn for two or three hours while your stomach struggles to unload itself, you're bound to wake up tired in the morning. (Besides, overloading your stomach at bedtime when muscles are inactive and circulation is at its slowest forces storage of calories and increases the fat content of the blood, contributing to a heart attack or stroke caused by clogging of arteries.)

The caffeine in coffee, tea, colas, and cocoa can prevent sleep by stimulating the nervous system. Usually, the stimulating effect of caffeine reaches its peak two to four hours after it is ingested. It's best, therefore, to avoid consumption of caffeine for at least seven hours before bedtime. This means that if you go to bed at 10 P.M., you should not have coffee or cola after 3 P.M.

Note: Even if coffee, tea, or cola does not keep you awake, there are other reasons why you should not drink them before going to bed. *The caffeine supplied by these beverages constricts blood vessels and increases blood fat.* Combine this with an increase in blood fat caused by overeating at bedtime and the slowdown in circulation that occurs during sleep, and the chances of heart attack or stroke are greatly increased in susceptible persons. Maybe this is one reason why most heart attacks occur during sleep.

Procedure 4: Control the environment of your bedroom. The conditions in your bedroom have much to do with how well you sleep. Temperature, for example, should be from 75 to 80 degrees, depending upon the relative humidity. Generally, a temperature of 78 degrees with a relative humidity of 45 percent would be comfortable for most people. Noises should be shut out as completely as possible. If you sleep during the day because of a night job, your room should be as free from daylight as possible.

Dress comfortably for bed. Sleepwear should not be so tight that it restricts movement or so loose that it tangles. Wear flannel in the winter and cotton in the summer. Make sure that heating or cooling units do not blow directly onto your bed.

Procedure 5: Supplement your diet with sleep-producing nutrients. Most people have learned from experience that drinking a glass of warm milk in the evening makes it easier to fall asleep at bedtime. It was dicovered recently that it is the amino acid *tryptophane* in milk that lulls the brain to sleep. Cheese, chicken, steak, tuna, peanut butter, and other protein-rich foods (except gelatin) also contain tryptophane. If you salt these foods, however, stimulation of your adrenal glands may offset the effect of the tryptophane.

Some doctors now prescribe 1,000 milligrams or more of tryptophane in pill form for persons suffering from insomnia.

Calcium and magnesium are believed to be natural tranquilizers. Many sleep-troubled celebrities take dolomite, a limestone supplement that contains the correct ratios of calcium and magnesium. (Milk is a good source of calcium.) Camomile tea is also a popular natural sedative.

Remember that a *deficiency* in calcium, magnesium, or B vitamins can contribute greatly to insomnia caused by nervous tension. So be sure to eat properly.

Try Sex or a Warm Bath

A warm tub bath at bedtime is a relaxing, sleep-inducing procedure. A *hot* bath, however, like a cold bath, may be stimulating rather than relaxing. Make sure that the water is comfortably warm.

Bedtime sex is a delightful tranquilizer, but only if the sex is satisfying. Sexual frustration caused by failure to climax as a result of inhibitions or improper techniques can play havoc with your nervous system. Read a good book on sex technique if your sex life is not helping you sleep at night.

HOW TO PREVENT FATIGUE
CAUSED BY ANEMIA

Anemia should always be suspected when there is unexplained fatigue. According the the U.S. Department of Agriculture (*Human Nutrition,* 1971), nutritional anemia is one of the most widely occurring deficiencies. *Iron defeciency* is the most common cause of nutrtional anemia. A survey conducted by the U.S. Department of Health, Education, and Welfare in 1968 revealed that the major nutritional deficiencies among low income families involved iron, Vitamins A, B_1, B_2, C, and folacin (folic acid). All of these nutrients play a role in the production of anemia.

Most nutritional deficiencies (according to prevailing standards) are the result of improper food selection. It has been estimated that one-fifth of U.S. diets do not provide "adequate nutrients" because of failure to eat the right foods. This means that many people do not eat well enough to take in *minimum* amounts of certain essential nutrients. Healthy persons (who are not pregnant or losing blood) who eat properly are not likely to develop any gross nutritional deficiencies within the allowances recommended by the National Research Council of the National Academy of Sciences. It seems likely, however, that some of the current recommended daily allowances are too low. So you should try to eat well enough to take in *more* of the essential nutrients than what is considered "adequate." This way, you'll be less likely to suffer from fatigue caused by a deficiency in iron or any other nutrient.

Actually, the body is very frugal with its iron. It normally retains iron released by worn-out blood cells and does not lose more than one milligram of iron a day except when blood is lost. This is why healthy persons may not need to ingest more than 18 milligrams of iron daily (of which only about 10 percent or less is absorbed). Persons who lose blood regularly (as in menstruation or from hemorrhoids) may need more iron than they can possibly get from food.

Anemia Should Be Treated by a Physician

Once iron-deficiency anemia occurs, for whatever reason, iron reserves throughout the body may be depleted. This means that large amounts of iron in supplement form are needed to restore reserves as well as to supply circulating blood cells. Too much iron, however, can be harmful, and there are many types of anemia that cannot be corrected by taking iron. This is why anemia should always be diagnosed and treated by a physician. When iron reserves have been restored and the red blood cells are carrying a full load of iron (as indicated by blood tests), the use of supplements may be discontinued. Adequate iron can then be obtained from food if there is no regular blood loss.

Food Sources of Iron

Whether you are anemic or not, you should make a special effort to eat iron-rich natural foods. Liver and blackstrap molasses are the richest sources of iron. (A generous serving of cooked calf liver supplies about 12 milligrams of iron. An equal amount of beef liver contains about seven milligrams of iron. One tablespoon of blackstrap molasses contains 3.2 milligrams of iron.) Meats, fish, oysters, egg yolk, green leafy vegetables, peas, beans, dried fruits, wheat germ, and whole-grain cereals are good sources of iron. (Remember that iron is more easily absorbed from animal products than from vegetables or cereals.)

Many processed foods are now enriched with iron, but such iron is difficult to absorb. You should not be eating processed foods anyway. *Natural* foods should be supplying the iron your body needs.

Folic acid supplied by green leafy vegetables is important in the treatment and prevention of anemia. According to the U.S. Department of Agriculture, "There is good evidence that folic acid deficiency may be a real problem in the U.S." One reason for this, of course, is that Americans are eating more processed foods and less fresh vegetables.

Dietary Supplements for Anemia

If you are a strict vegetarian and you do not eat animal products, you should supplement your diet with Vitamin B_{12}. Vegetables do not contain Vitamin B_{12}, and their folic acid content tends to mask the symptoms of a Vitamin B_{12} deficiency. If you do not eat meat, try to include other animal products in your diet. Milk, cheese, and eggs, for example, contain Vitamin B_{12}. Persons suffering from pernicious anemia because of an inability to absorb Vitamin B_{12} may have to receive regular injections of the vitamin from a physician.

Iron-deficiency anemia in older persons who do not have enough stomach acid to facilitate absorption of iron can benefit from taking betaine hydrochloride tablets with meals. This will supply the acid needed for absorption of iron. Ascorbic acid (Vitamin C) taken with meals will also aid absorption of iron.

If you are on a low-calorie diet, or if you have reason to suspect that you are anemic or might become anemic, go ahead and supplement your diet with 18 to 25 milligrams of ferrous sulfate or ferrous gluconate. But be sure to have your blood tested occasionally. When the hemoglobin (iron and protein) in your red blood cells reaches a level of 15 grams per 100 milliliters of blood, you won't need additional iron. (Fifteen grams of hemoglobin contain about 50 milligrams of iron. The total amount of blood in the body contains about four grams of iron.)

Whenever a blood test reveals that you are anemic in spite of eating properly and taking an iron supplement, follow your doctor's instructions and see a good hematologist. It might be necessary to take as much as 300 milligrams of ferrous sulfate or ferrous gluconate three times a day for awhile to correct severe iron-deficiency anemia. (Remember that only *part* of ferrous sulfate or ferrous gluconate is actually iron. Taking 300 milligrams of either of these supplements three times a day would supply only about 290 milligrams of iron a day, of which only about 20 or 30 milligrams will be absorbed. This is still a huge dose of iron, however, and must be taken only under the supervision of a physician.) Types of anemia that cannot be corrected by taking iron or eating iron-rich foods may require other forms of treatment.

SUMMARY

1. Chronic fatigue may be a warning that you are doing something wrong in caring for your body.

2. Hypoglycemia triggered by excessive consumption of sugar and white-flour products is a common cause of chronic fatigue.

3. The best treatment for hypoglycemia (low blood sugar) is to eat a variety of fresh, natural foods at mealtime and then snack on protein-rich natural foods between meals.

4. The caffeine in coffee, tea, colas, and cocoa can trigger hypoglycemia in susceptible persons by stimulating the adrenal glands.

5. Brewer's yeast and desiccated liver supply B vitamins and other nutrients needed to combat fatigue.

6. Unrelieved stress and tension can lead to depression as well as to chronic fatigue.

7. Try to end each day with activities that relieve your mind and induce relaxation.

8. Make sure that you do everything you can to get adequate sleep each night in a controlled environment.

9. You must make a special effort to eat iron-rich natural foods if you want to prevent the development of iron-deficiency anemia.

10. Since there are many types of anemia, some of which cannot be corrected by taking iron, treatment of any form of anemia should be supervised by a physician.

10

Tips from Celebrities on Preparing Basic Foods in a Health-Building Program

In practically every chapter of this book, something was said about the importance of good nutrition. You know that you have to eat right to be slim and energetic. You need high-quality protein for strong muscles. You *must* have optimum amounts of vitamins and minerals to prevent disease and infection. You learned in Chapter 8 that many of the leading causes of death are the result of bad eating habits. Everyone knows that you have to be healthy to have attractive skin and hair, and so on.

Every aspect of your body-improvement program must be backed up by good nutrition. You already know what foods you must eat. Unless these foods are properly prepared, however, they won't supply you with adequate nourishment. That's what this chapter is all about—how to cook or prepare fiber-rich, low-fat *natural* foods so that they do not lose precious nutrients.

When *Yvonne De Carlo* was asked how she stayed so fit and beautiful, she replied: "Food has a great deal to do with it. And although I do not live solely on health foods, I am a great cook."

COOKING IS A GREAT HOBBY

Healthful cooking can be a useful and interesting hobby. Every health-conscious celebrity we know is knowledgeable about selecting and preparing foods. *Most of them are good cooks.* You should be a good cook, too, if you want to do as much for your body as you can. You don't have to cook like *Dinah Shore* or *Suzanne Somers,* both of whom are gourmet cooks, but you should know the *basic rules* of cooking. If you prepare your foods properly so that they retain fiber as well as nutrients, you won't have to eat so much to satisfy your hunger and to get the nutrients you need for good health. Improperly prepared foods *always* lose vitamins and minerals, but they do not

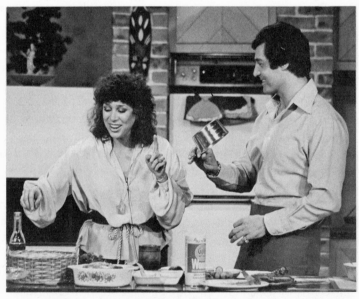

Actress Liz Torres tells Peter Lupus that it's all right to cook food if you do not use an excessive amount of heat or water.

lose calories. In fact, some cooking methods *increase* the calorie content of food while lowering its nutritional value.

To get the most out of the food you eat without getting too many calories, it's essential that you know something about cooking or preparing foods. Even if you do not cook yourself, you should be able to tell others how your meals should be prepared. Super-energetic *Liz Torres* attributes her inexhaustible energy—and her success in films— to the fact that she is particular about how her foods are prepared.

To Cook or Not to Cook . . .

Many foods should not be cooked. Fruits and nuts, for example, should always be eaten raw. Many vegetables, such as lettuce, tomatoes, cucumbers, are best eaten raw. Some vegetables, such as cauliflower, carrots, and rutabaga, may yield more nutrients when they are cooked a little. There are a few vegetables that must always be cooked. Certain beans, for example, can be toxic when eaten raw. A vegetable that does not have a pleasant flavor when raw may be delicious when properly cooked.

Meat, fish, eggs, and poultry should *always* be cooked to destroy any bacteria or parasites they might contain. Since these foods are eaten primarily for the protein and iron they supply, cooking them does not diminish their nutritional value.

In this chapter you'll learn everything you need to know about cooking and preparing foods. Male or female, you should not hesitate to put on an apron or go into the kitchen. Food preparation is as much a part of the *Peter Lupus Body-Improvement Program* as exercise. In fact, the studio set of "Peter Lupus' Body Shop" television show included a kitchen where guest experts and celebrities could demonstrate preparation of their favorite food or beverage.

So don't skip this chapter just because you do not do your own cooking. After you read this chapter, you'll either do your own cooking or you'll tell someone else how to do it.

Don't Fry with Fat!

The first rule of healthful cooking, as far as we are concerned, is that *you should not fry foods in grease or oil.* In addition to adding extra calories, fats and oils that are heated above a certain temperature (419 degrees Fahrenheit for 15 minutes or longer) are broken down to form a toxic substance. Furthermore, excessive use of fats and oils of any kind may contribute to the development of cancer.

If you do fry something occasionally, use fresh vegetable oil and keep the temperature down so that the oil does not smoke. (When any cooking fat begins to smoke, it is being overheated.) Vegetable oils (except olive oil) and hydrogenated shortenings have a higher smoking temperature than lard and other forms of animal fat and will therefore withstand higher temperatures. But remember that heating vegetable oil destroys its essential fatty acids (those you need for good health). When vegetable oil is used over and over in deep frying, the smoking temperature becomes lower and lower. The oil literally decomposes each time it is heated. *Don't use cooking fats or oils more than once.* Fry as little as you can—and use fresh vegetable oil each time.

Beware of Charcoal Grilling

We don't want to be party poopers, but we have to tell you that we do not recommend charcoal grilling. Meat that has been charred by direct contact with smoke and flame contains cancer-causing substances that are formed by heat and deposited by smoke. Simply frying a hamburger may form carcinogens on the surface of the meat. When a hamburger is burned by fire and blackened by smoke, it is even more carcinogenic.

There are many ways to cook meats safely. Baking or broiling meats, for example, so that the meat is not in direct contact with the source of the heat, will not result in burning or overheating. You'll learn more about how to cook meats later in this chapter.

Stir-Frying Is Okay

The only exception to the rule about no frying is stir-frying—or sauteing. This method of cooking can be used when you want to barely cook small pieces of meat and vegetables in a short period of

time. The food to be cooked is cut into small pieces and placed in a pan containing a small amount of hot vegetable oil (no more than two tablespoons). You simply stir the food until it is coated with oil and cooked just enough to eat. Very few nutrients are lost in this method of cooking, and the natural taste and color of the food are retained. The small amount of oil used will seal in nutrients without any harmful effects, since there is no overheating.

If you do not want to use oil in stir-frying, you can use water. Just keep adding a little water or bouillon while stirring the food in a hot pan. Stir-frying with water, however, may result in loss of more nutrients than when sauteing with oil.

Actress *Janet Du Bois* proved to us that simple cooking methods are best by quickly preparing a delicious vegetable dish in the "Body Shop" kitchen. "The best way to cook vegetables," she said, "is to do as little cooking as possible."

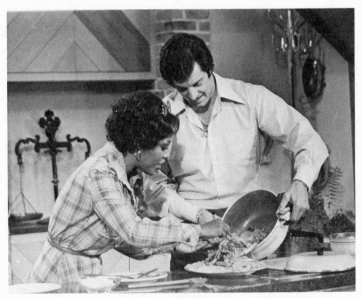

Janet DuBois, co-star of the television series "Good Times," demonstrates preparation of a vegetable dish made up entirely of fresh vegetables.

The *best* way to cook vegetables is to steam them or cook them in only a small amount of water. Before you begin cooking, however, there are a few basic rules you should follow, no matter how you cook your food.

BASIC RULES FOR HEALTHFUL COOKING

Regardless of the type of food you're cooking, you should use as little heat, water, and time as possible to get the job done. The less surface area of the food exposed to air the better. Vitamin C, all of the B vitamins, and some minerals (such as potassium) are soluble in water, and the more water used the greater the loss of these nutrients. (Boiled or processed foods which have been salted are high in sodium and low in potassium, contributing to the development of high blood pressure, water retention, and other problems.)

Heat and oxygen also destroy nutrients, particularly Vitamin C, Vitamin A, and thiamine. Obviously, the longer a food is exposed to all the factors involved in cooking the greater the loss of nutrients. This doesn't mean, however, that you should quit cooking. It means that you should always cook your foods *properly*—and never more than necessary.

Cutting of foods should also be kept to a minimum. The more a food is cut the greater the surface area exposed to the destructive effect of oxygen and water. It will, of course, occasionally be necessary to cut foods into fairly small peices to shorten cooking time, especially in stir-frying. But don't cut any more than necessary. You should *never* shred a food. Many foods, especially vegetables, can be cooked without any cutting whatsoever. Potatoes, for example, can be baked or boiled whole. You should do everything you can to avoid breaking open the reservoir of nutrients inside a vegetable during cooking.

Cook Fresh Foods Daily

Even if you cook your foods properly, they will lose nutrients when stored overnight or longer. Reheating also results in loss of nutrients. Cooked vegetables reheated after two or three days in a refrigerator, for example, will contain only one-third to one-half as much Vitamin C as when freshly prepared. *Always try to cook your foods fresh each day,* especially in the case of vegetables. If you do keep cooked vegetables for several hours, keep them covered to exclude light and air. Exposing a food to light results in destruction of riboflavin, one of the B vitamins, while exposure to light and oxygen destroys Vitamin C.

Fats and oils turn rancid when stored too long. You should *never* consume rancid fats and oils. Rancidity means that oxygen has destroyed the fat's essential fatty acids and Vitamin A as well as their protective Vitamin E. Besides, rancid fat contains peroxides and other substances that may be harmful to your body.

Simple cooking methods are best. Broiling meats, baking potatoes, steaming vegetables, and serving fruits (and some vegetables) raw is much more healthful than gourmet cooking methods that disguise the true taste and appearance of foods. Actually, simple cooking methods that bring out the natural flavor of food have much more to offer your taste buds (and your body) than more destructive methods of cooking. Don't ever feel sorry for yourself when you sit down for a meal consisting of plain, natural foods that have been prepared in a simple manner. You are way ahead of the person who prepares fancy meals that are loaded with calories and deficient in nutrients.

HOW TO COOK VEGETABLES PROPERLY

Did you know that the outer dark-green leaves of lettuce, cabbage, collards, broccoli, and other greens have more Vitamin A than the inner leaves? Don't discard the outer leaves just because they are coarse. And don't discard the fibrous core of cabbage, which is rich in Vitamin C. Vegetables are an important source of the fiber you need for good health. You may even eat the fibrous stems and midribs of leafy vegetables if they are not too tough to chew. Cooking a vegetable will soften fibrous ribs and break down their cellulose enough to release nutrients. Remember, however, that a vegetable should never be cooked until it is mushy. Any vegetable is adequately cooked when it is soft enough to penetrate with a fork. A properly cooked vegetable will, in fact, be a little crispy, indicating that fiber as well as nutrients have been retained.

The skins of such vegetables as carrots, potatoes, and tomatoes are also rich in fiber and nutrients. Don't ever peel a vegetable unless the skin is not edible. Eat the whole vegetable whenever possible. You need plenty of fiber in your diet to control your body weight and to prevent the development of colon cancer.

Raw vegetables, in which cellulose has not been softened by cooking, are especially rich in fiber. *Eat something raw every day.* Every time you prepare a fresh vegetable for cooking, put aside a portion for use in a raw salad. Salads are popular among actors who must watch their weight and look their best to fit their roles. "Wonder Woman" *Lynda Carter,* for example, reported that her *main meal* each day is a big salad dressed with sesame oil and fresh lemon juice. Lynda is five feet eight inches tall and weighs 122 pounds—and she's

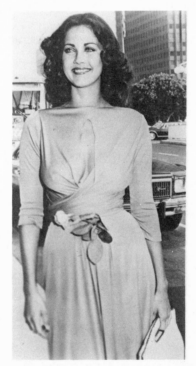

TV Wonder Woman Lynda Carter keeps her "Miss World" figure by selecting and preparing her foods carefully on the set as well as at home.

beautiful! "Captain" *Gavin MacLeod* of "Love Boat," who reduced his body weight from 265 pounds to 184 pounds (see Chapter 11), also puts salads first on his diet. "For lunch," he said, "I'll have a lettuce and tomato salad, with a tablespoon of oil and vinegar. In the afternoon, I'll have an apple, an orange, a peach, or some other kind of fruit. Dinner, which is my big meal, starts with a salad, which is a *large* salad."

Even if you cook your vegetables properly, be sure to eat some of them raw if you want to eat like the stars.

Steaming Is the Best Way to Cook a Vegetable

Steaming a vegetable minimizes its contact with heat, air, and water, thus conserving nutrients. Just place the vegetable in a covered collander that is resting over a pot of boiling water. The steam passing up through the vegetables will do the cooking. Do not cut the vegetable into pieces any smaller than necessary to permit cooking.

You can also steam vegetables by cooking them in a pot that contains only enough water to prevent scorching. Bring the water to a boil before dropping in the vegetables and then cover the pot with a tight-fitting lid to hold in the steam. The steam will displace the air and reduce oxidation of nutrients. Use low heat, and remove the vegetables from the pot as soon as they are done enough to eat. Vegetables that are only slightly cooked have a mild, sweet flavor, but when overcooked they may develop a strong, undesirable flavor. (It is not as easy to overcook a vegetable when steaming as when boiling.)

How to Boil a Vegetable

You shouldn't boil vegetables very often. Boiling is occasionally necessary, however. To get the best results, put only enough water in the pot to equal about one-third the volume of the vegetable you have prepared for cooking. Bring the water to a boil *before* dropping in the vegetable and putting on the lid. Frozen vegetables should be kept frozen until they are dropped into the boiling water.

Leave the skins on carrots and potatoes when you boil them, and cook them *whole* whenever possible. This will help prevent the release of water-soluble vitamins and minerals into the cooking water. Potatoes boiled whole in their skin, for example, retain practically all of their Vitamin C, thiamine, and other nutrients. When cut vegetables are boiled, nutrients seep into the water.

Dried peas and beans (legumes) must always be boiled to rehydrate them. First drop the legumes into a pot of boiling water and cook them for two minutes. Then remove the pot from the stove and let the legumes soak in the cooking water for one hour before finishing the cooking. This procedure will conserve nutrients as well as eliminate the customary 15 hours of cold-water soaking. (Dried legumes cook much faster in *soft* water. A small amount of sodium bicarbonate softens the hard water but may increase the loss of B vitamins during cooking.)

Get a Health-High on Pot Liquor

Water (pot liquor) left over from boiling vegetables or beans is loaded with water-soluble nutrients. If you don't season cooked vegetables or beans with oil or animal fat, you may use the leftover water as a beverage or a soup. Pot liquor that isn't greasy will not require reheating before consumption. (You should not drink greasy pot liquor, hot or cold!)

If you like, you can season cooked vegetables with a small amount of salt or bouillon, which will, in turn, flavor leftover water. If you're on a low-sodium diet and you cannot use salt or bouillon (which is usually salty), and you feel that a vegetable needs seasoning, try using chives, onions, green pepper, garlic, celery seeds, and other herbs and spices. Remember, however, that a taste for salt and other forms of seasoning is cultivated. You can learn to appreciate the delicious natural flavor of a properly cooked vegetable that has not been seasoned.

Don't Be Fooled by Color

Many cooks add baking soda to cooking water to preserve the color of green vegetables. Vinegar is sometimes used to preserve the color of red vegetables cooked in hard water. Lemon juice or white vinegar added to cooking water helps retain the color of white vegetables. Such cooking techniques make a vegetable more attractive in appearance, but they detract from nutritional value. Baking soda, for example, destroys Vitamin C and tends to produce soft, mushy vegetables. Adding vinegar to cooking water may contribute to destruction of nutrients by prolonging cooking time, and so on.

If you cook your vegetables properly (with as little heat, water, and time as possible), they will retain most of their color as well as their flavor and nutrients. When you want brightly colored vegetables for special occasions, try cooking (steaming or boiling) the vegetables in milk. Simmer each vegetable in milk heated to about 200 degrees Fahrenheit. Be sure to use the leftover cooking milk as a soup or as a sauce.

You can preserve the color of cut apples, bananas, and other fruits by dripping them in the juice of a lemon, an orange, a grapefruit, or a pineapple. The Vitamin C in acid fruit juices is a natural antioxidant and will prevent the discoloration caused by exposure to oxygen.

Potatoes Are Special

The best way to cook potatoes is to bake them. If the potato is properly cleaned beforehand, you may eat the entire potato, jacket and all. Most of the flavor, the nutrients, and the fiber are in the jacket. The habit many people have of scooping out the soft center of the potato and leaving a hollowed-out potato on their plate is wasteful and unwise. If any member of your family leaves a potato jacket on the dinner table, put the jacket back in the oven and brown it. A crisply done jacket seasoned with a little salt is delicious.

When you bake potatoes in their jackets, cook them for about 50 minutes at 400 degrees Fahrenheit. When they are soft enough to penetrate with a fork, they are done enough. Pricking the skin of a potato before baking will prevent splitting by allowing steam to escape. If a potato seems to be dry after baking, you can moisten it with pot liquor left over from cooked vegetables. Or you can use a low-calorie buttermilk dressing.

To make a buttermilk dressing, mix two-thirds of a cup of cottage cheese with one-fourth of a cup of buttermilk. Add one-half teaspoon of lemon juice and mix in a blender. Serve immediately or chill in a refrigerator. A chilled dresssing is great for cooling a hot potato. Plain yogurt (sometimes mixed with cottage cheese) is often used as a dressing for baked potatoes.

The potato is *Lucille Ball's* favorite vegetable. "I *love* potatoes," she told us. "I can eat them 18 times a day, but I only eat them three times a week . . . . Years ago, when I was a kid living in New York, I was poor—and I mean *poor.* If I was asked out to dinner I would put butter on a bun, cover it with a napkin, and slip it into my purse for breakfast. At that time, I had friends—a married couple—who were as poor as I was. She worked in a bookstore and he stayed home and tried to write. One night I was asked over to their house for dinner. They served five

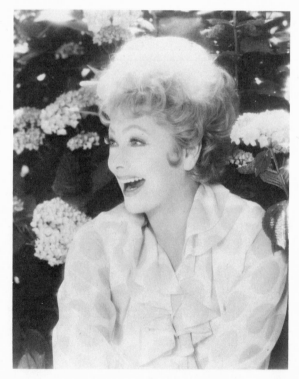

*Comedienne Lucille Ball remains beautiful and vivacious
at the age of 69 because of good health habits.*

different kinds of potatoes with wine—nothing else. I never had a better dinner in my life!"

Potatoes are not nearly as fattening as most people think. A baked potato, for example, contains fewer calories than a serving of beef. (One *lean* hamburger patty, broiled, contains *twice* as many calories as one medium potato.)

Note: You can also bake corn. Leave the shuck on the corn and bake for 10 to 12 minutes at 400 degrees Fahrenheit or until the shuck begins to turn brown. Corn cooked in this manner is much more delicious and nutritious than boiled corn.

THE INSIDE SCOOP ON FRUITS,
JUICES, AND SALADS

The cellulose in raw fruits and vegetables supplies fiber that may be more healthful than the bran supplied by whole-grain products. Cellulose holds moisture in your bowels and provides a good environment for the growth of friendly bacteria. It also serves as a broom in sweeping your bowels clean. Remember, however, that cooking fruits and vegetables softens the cellulose and breaks it down so that it loses its straw-like texture. This is one reason why you should eat vegetables raw whenever possible. Fruits, of course, should *always* be eaten raw—and they should be eaten *whole.*

Except on special occasions when you need a fruit-juice beverage, you should never squeeze a fruit for juice and then throw away the pulp. The juice will contain most of the Vitamin C, Vitamin A, and potassium of the fruit, but the pulp contains valuable fiber as well as nutrients. When you have a choice, eat the pulp of the fruit—and the skin, too, if it is clean (unwaxed and unsprayed) and edible. The bulk supplied by cellulose will help satisfy your appetite so that you'll eat less of other more-fattening foods.

When impersonator *Rich Little* reduced his body weight 27 pounds, he did it by eating salads for bulk so that he could cut back on other foods. "They're the greatest thing in the world for bulk," he said. Fruits also supply bulk, but since they also contain fructose (sugar), you should not depend solely upon fruits for bulk. Combining raw vegetables with fruits is best. When you squeeze a fruit for juice, you concentrate its sugar as well as eliminate its bulk. If you use a blender to make fruit drinks, use the whole fruit so that the pulp of the fruit becomes a part of the drink.

The Special Benefits of Fruit

Since fruits are low in sodium and high in potassium, they are ideal foods for persons on a low-sodium diet. If you have high blood pressure, or if you are taking diuretics, you should eat plenty of fresh fruit (or drink it from a blender).

Be sure to eat a *variety* of fresh fruits. Some contain more Vitamin A or Vitamin C than others. The citrus fruits, such as oranges, grapefruit, lemons, limes, and tangerines, are highest in Vitamin C. Guava, a popular Hawaiian fruit, is also a rich source of Vitamin C. Strawberries compare favorably with citrus fruits as a source of Vitamin C. Berries contain Vitamin C, but they require special handling and lose nutrients easily. Fruits highest in Vitamin A include apricots, yellow-fleshed peaches, deeply-colored cantaloupes, mangoes, papayas, and other yellow fruits.

Try to eat whatever fruit is in season. Fresh fruits provide a taste treat as well as a body treatment. In addition to providing essential nutrients, fruits supply pectin that absorbs and eliminates toxins from the intestinal tract. Acid fruits aid absorption of iron and calcium. Figs, pineapple, and papaya contain enzymes that aid digestion of protein. Prunes and melons aid elimination. *Every fruit has something special to offer.* Be sure to have fresh fruit with each meal, whatever is in season.

"Angel" *Jaclyn Smith* cultivated a taste for fruit-and-vegetable salads after moving to the West Coast. "The fresh fruits and vegetables there are just beautiful," she observed, "and they are always available."

If you are fortunate enough to live in an area where fresh fruits and vegetables are plentiful, be sure to take advantage of your good luck.

Whenever possible, *finish a meal with fresh fruit.* Cheese and fruit make a satisfying dessert. (*Joan Rivers'* favorite dessert is cheese and an apple.) If you must have something sweeter, eat dates, raisins, or dried figs. Dried fruits are good sources of calcium and iron. Raisins can be used to sweeten (and enrich) cereals and other foods.

HOW TO GET MAXIMUM
NOURISHMENT FROM MEAT

We eat meats primarily for the protein they supply. Since meat is the most expensive food we eat, you'll be pleased to learn that *you can get just as much protein from cheaper cuts of meat as from more expensive cuts.* The only difference is that the cheaper cuts may be a little tougher. One reason for this is that cheaper meat usually comes from a portion of the animal where the muscle is denser from more frequent use. This may also mean, however, that the meat has *less fat,* which makes the meat more healthful.

Many tender and more expensive cuts of meat contain less muscle and more fat. Prime rib, for example, is juicy and tender because it is loaded with fat. Since it's best to cut down on your intake of animal fat as much as possible to protect your health, consumption of fat meat should be kept to a minimum. For this reason, it's often best to select the cheaper cut of meat, even if it is a little tougher. Besides, it's good exercise for your teeth to chew tough meat. If the meat is properly cooked, it won't be too tough to eat. And if you can swallow it, you can digest it.

The nutritional value of protein is not greatly affected by cooking. How you cook a meat, therefore, is not as important as how you cook a vegetable. The primary reasons for cooking meats are to destroy bacteria and parasites and to improve taste. You should, however, use cooking methods that conserve B vitamins and reduce fat content. Also, if you use the correct cooking method for the type of meat you have, the meat will be more tender. Overcooking a meat will toughen it as well as destroy B vitamins, particularly thiamine.

Pork is rich in thiamine, but since it often contains parasites, it should always be cooked until it is *well done.* Don't worry about conserving thiamine when you cook pork. Just make sure that it isn't pink when you eat it.

Of all the meats, liver is richest in nutrients. In addition to protein and B vitamins, liver is rich in iron and Vitamin B_{12}; it also contains

Vitamin C. Liver should be cooked, but not too much if you want to conserve its nutrients.

The Meat Cut Determines the Cooking Method

Generally, the cheaper, tougher (more muscular) meats should be cooked in the presence of moisture, as in boiling, braising, stewing, or simmering. This will make the meat more tender by dissolving the collagen that holds the muscle fibers together. Meat will lose B vitamins in the presence of moisture, however, so the broth or meat stock should be saved for use in soups. Chill the stock before using so that you can skim off and discard the hard fat.

Fatty or more expensive meats (or meats from young animals) are best cooked with dry heat. Baking, roasting, or broiling, for example, are popular methods of dry-heat cooking. Meats that can be cooked with dry heat usually do not need to be cooked as long as leaner, tougher meats. So be careful not to overcook if you want tender meat.

It might be wise to collect the meat drippings when you cook meats with dry heat. If you chill the drippings and skim off the hard fat, the vitamin-rich water you have left can be reheated and poured over meat to improve taste and to restore lost moisture and nutrients.

How to Slow-Cook Meat
with Roasting or Dry Cooking

Oven roasting is the best way to dry-cook a large piece of meat. First trim away all surface fat except for a thin layer. Then place the meat on a rack in a shallow pan (fat side up so that the meat will be self basting). Heat the oven to 325 degrees Fahrenheit and roast the meat to the desired degree of doneness. Remember that meat cooked slowly at a lower temperature is juicier and more tender than meat cooked rapidly at a high temperature.

Don't salt meat until *after* it has been cooked. Salting the meat while it is cooking will draw out its juices.

If you have a meat thermometer, insert the thermometer into the thickest portion of the meat where it won't touch the bone. The temperature in the center of the meat will accurately reflect the degree of doneness. When the temperature reaches 170 degrees Fahrenheit, for example, the meat is well done. A temperature of 160 degrees is medium, while a temperature of 140 degrees is rare. (Generally, it takes about 45 minutes per pound to cook beef well done.) Pork should be cooked until it is no longer pink or until its internal temperature is 185 degrees Fahrenheit.

How to Broil Meat
for Quick Cooking

When you want to cook smaller pieces of meat (or poultry) quickly, try broiling. Place the meat on a rack in a broiler pan so that the meat will be three to six inches from the source of heat, depending upon how brown you want your meat to be. When one side has browned, sprinkle the browned surface with salt and then turn the meat over and brown the other side. It's best not to preheat the oven when you broil meat, and you should leave the oven door *open.*

When you broil chicken, you'll have to decide for yourself whether you want to remove the skin or leave it on. Cooking chicken in its skin keeps it moist and tender. But since most of the fat of chicken is in the skin, you should not eat the skin. If you like your chicken brown and you do not want to eat the skin, you should remove the skin *before* cooking. Chicken browned without its skin is a little tougher, but it is practically zero in fat.

You can also broil fish. But remember that it takes only about five minutes to cook fish adequately. When fish is creamy white and easily flaked with a fork, it is cooked enough.

Recommended reading: *Food,* published by the U.S. Department of Agriculture, and *Let's Cook it Right* (New American Library), by Adelle Davis.

BALANCING PROTEIN WITH
WHOLE-GRAIN CEREALS AND BREADS

Whole-grain cereals and breads are nutritional bargains. Rich in protein, minerals, and B vitamins, they also supply fiber and Vitamin E. Breads and cereals made from milled grains, however, do not contain the nutrients and the fiber found in whole grains. Super-nutritious wheat germ, for example, is removed from wheat in the milling process. The miller's bran that everyone is now adding to cereals and other foods has also been removed from wheat. Many nutrients are destroyed in the milling process. When you have a choice, always select whole-grain products.

Although whole-grain breads and cereals are rich in protein, they do not contain a *complete* protein. This means that you should combine whole-grain products with other foods to form a complete protein that your body can use to build tissue. Using milk on cereal, peanut butter on bread, cheese with grits, and so on, will combine amino acids (the building blocks of protein) to form a complete protein. Grains and beans used together, as in rice and beans, provide a complete vegetable protein. Unless you are a knowledgeable vegetarian, however, and you know how to combine foods to form a complete protein, you should not attempt to get all of your protein from grains and vegetables. You should concentrate on getting your protein from animal products (not necessarily meat) and then use whole-grain products for their fiber and vitamin-and-mineral content. The protein supplied by grains will then complement your other sources of protein.

Gloria Swanson is a knowledgeable vegetarian who manages to stay healthy without eating meat. "The best diet I've found," she says, "consists of nuts, fresh fruits, and fresh vegetables." Few people, however, are knowledgeable enough about diet to get by on a strict vegetarian diet of fruits, nuts, vegetables, and grains without suffering a deficiency. This is why persons who do not eat red meat are usually advised to include fish, poultry, or animal products (such as milk, eggs, and cheese) in their diet. *Paul Michael Glaser,* for example, has salads for lunch and supper, but he often includes fish or chicken to assure an adequate supply of protein. *Dennis Weaver* substitutes cheese for meat in his diet. *Daryl and Toni Tennille* do not eat meat, but they include milk, eggs, and milk products in their diet.

Many Hollywood stars are now switching to a vegetarian-type diet that eliminates red meat but includes fish and poultry or milk, eggs, and cheese. *Englebert Humperdinck* recently made such a change. "I stopped eating steaks and most red meats," he revealed. "I eat mostly fish and chicken now, with a lot of fresh vegetables." *Carol Burnett* eats raw or lightly cooked vegetables in a balanced diet that does not include red meat. *Carol Channing* eats organically grown fruits and vegetables in a diet that includes fish and such animal products as cheese in order to balance the protein in her diet. When she does eat beef, it's always organically fed beef from her own West Coast farm.

We recommend that the average person eat a balanced diet made up of a variety of foods to guard against possible deficiencies. If you don't eat red meat (or the flesh of any living creature), you should eat such animal products as cheese or eggs, even if you eat a combination of protein-rich grains, nuts, and legumes. The Vitamin B_{12} you need for good health is provided exclusively by foods of animal origin. The bacteria in your intestinal tract manufactures some B_{12}, and traces of the vitamin are found in wheat germ, brewer's yeast,

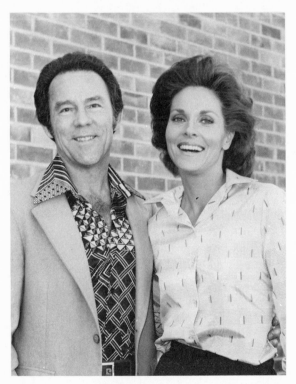

Lee Meriwether, co-star of the "Barnaby Jones" television series and a former "Miss America," explains to Dr. Samuel Homola how jogging and good nutrition keep her physically fit.

and soy beans. But if you don't eat animal products, you should supplement your diet with Vitamin B$_{12}$.

Whatever type of diet you follow, be sure to *include generous amounts of whole-grain products.* You can choose from whole-wheat flour, brown rice, dark rye flour, whole-ground cornmeal, oatmeal, and breads and cereals made from these grains. It's all right to eat sandwiches when they are made with whole-grain bread. You can, in fact, make a meal out of a good sandwich. When we interviewed *Lee Meriwether* over lunch at a health food restaurant, she ate tuna fish on stone-ground whole-wheat bread, dressed with melted Cheddar cheese, fresh tomatoes, lettuce, and bean sprouts. Her beverage was a mixture of pineapple juice and coconut juice.

Try to be consistent in eating properly. If you cannot buy a good lunch when you are away from home, take your lunch with you, especially if you eat sandwiches.

Watch for Gluten Allergy!

If you happen to be allergic to gluten, a protein substance found in wheat, rye, oats, and barley, you may have to avoid all whole-grain products except those made from corn and rice. Flour for bread can be obtained from corn, rice, soybeans, and potatoes.

Gluten allergy, or celiac disease, is a form of diarrhea that is characterized by foamy, light-colored stools. Remember that any product containing wheat or rye protein contains gluten. Read labels carefully. The white flour in most processed foods, for example, is usually made from wheat. If you have a gluten problem, ask your doctor for a gluten-gliaden-free diet.

Choosing a Cereal

There are now many good whole-grain cereals on the market. Shredded wheat, granola, grape nuts, oatmeal, and brown rice, for example, are commonly available. If honey-sweetened granola cereals are too sweet for you, you can mix in a little shredded wheat. Unsweetened cereals can be sweetened with fresh or dried fruit.

You can add miller's bran to your cereal for additional fiber if you like. A teaspoon of brewer's yeast powder and a couple tablespoons of wheat germ mixed into a bowl of cereal will boost your intake of B vitamins, iron, Vitamin E, and magnesium.

If you cook whole-grain cereals, such as oats or brown rice, use only as much water as the cereal will absorb. This will assure retention of water-soluble vitamins and minerals. Don't buy the quick-cooking variety of cereals. Such cereals have been precooked or processed and stripped of fiber and nutrients. It takes longer to cook natural, whole-grain cereals, but the nutrients you get are well worth the effort. Besides, when the protective coating of a grain is removed, the grain loses more nutrients to heat, light, air, and water. Simply washing white rice, for example, removes 25 percent of its thiamine, compared with only 10 percent when washing brown rice. (You should not wash any grain before cooking unless absolutely necessary.)

Recipes for Homemade
Whole-Grain Bread

Everyone should experience the pleasure of eating homemade whole-wheat bread. You can get whole-wheat flour in most grocery stores.

Here's a recipe for whole-wheat bread that anyone can follow successfully:

Mix 3 cups of warm water with ½ cup of honey and 2 packages of baker's yeast. Allow this mixture to stand for 5 minutes or longer and then add 5 cups of unsifted stone-ground whole-wheat flour.

Beat this mixture by hand 100 times or more.

Then add 2 or 3 cups more of whole-wheat flour (or enough to make the dough stiff) and 1 scant tablespoon of salt.

Knead the dough until it is smooth and elastic, adding enough flour to prevent sticking.

Place the dough in an oiled bowl, in a warm place, and let the dough rise until it doubles in bulk.

Knead the dough back to its original size and place it in two 1½-pound loaf pans that have been greased with margarine.

Let the dough rise until it reaches the top of the pan before placing it in the oven.

Bake in a preheated oven at 350 degrees Fahrenheit for about 60 minutes or until the bread is browned.

Bread baked to a medium brownness loses about 20 percent of its thiamine. Toasting a slice of bread reduces its thiamine content by 15 to 20 percent—and the darker the toast the greater the loss. Don't toast bread with the idea of improving its nutritional value. If you do toast bread, toast it lightly.

Treat Yourself with Corn Bread

Old-fashioned corn bread is nutritious as well as delicious. Eat it often. If you cannot eat wheat bread because of a gluten allergy, you can eat corn bread.

Here's a simple recipe for corn pone:

Mix 3 cups of white cornmeal with ½ teaspoon of salt.

Then pour in ¼ cup of corn oil and several cups of boiling water. Mix and form into patties.

Bake in a 350-degree (Fahrenheit) oven for about 50 minutes.

If you like, you can enhance the taste and protein content of corn bread by adding one-third cup of sesame seeds.

Katherine Helmond of the television series "Soap" is a health-food advocate who has her own special recipe for corn bread. "I'm sure that much of my success as an actress comes from my devotion to health food," she claims. "It keeps my weight down, my health good, and gives me a high energy level."

Here is her recipe for "wheat germ corn bread":

1 cup whole wheat flour

1 cup wheat germ

one-third cup honey

1 cup stone-ground cornmeal

5 teaspoons baking powder

1 teaspoon salt

1 ½ cups milk

3 large eggs

one-third cup soy margarine

These ingredients are mixed and sprinkled with sesame seeds or sunflower seeds before baking until done (about 45 minutes) in an oven heated to 350 degrees Fahrenheit.

With a little imagination, you can alter any bread recipe to include your favorite flour, grains, or seeds.

MILK, CHEESE, AND EGGS

Milk and milk products normally provide about two-thirds of the total amount of calcium in our diet and more than a fifth of our protein. They also supply riboflavin and Vitamin A. When milk is skimmed, however, or has had its fat (and cholesterol) removed, the Vitamin A is removed. Cottage cheese and other products made from skimmed milk are also low in Vitamin A.

A glass of skimmed milk has only about half as many calories as a glass of whole milk. This is one reason why skimmed milk is so popular. But unless you are on a reducing diet or you have a blood cholesterol problem, you should not completely eliminate whole milk or its products from your diet. Cheddar cheese, for example, is rich in Vitamin A as well as calcium and protein.

Many adults do not have the digestive enzyme they need to digest lactose or milk sugar. As a result, they suffer from gas pains and other digestive disturbances when they consume milk or its products. Fermenting milk to make cottage cheese, yogurt, or buttermilk will solve this problem by converting lactose to lactic acid. Enzymes are now available in tablet form for persons who have trouble digesting milk sugar. You simply take the tablets when you drink milk or eat milk products.

If you buy milk that must be stored for several days, be sure to keep it in an airtight container in a dark place. Exposing milk to light results in loss of riboflavin, an important nutrient in milk.

Eggs Are Good for You!

The protein supplied by egg white is the best protein you can get for your body—and eggs are *rich* in protein. Two eggs contain about 12 grams of high-quality protein. They are also rich in iron, Vitamins A, D, E, K, and all the B vitamins. If you are on a low-fat diet, egg yolk can supply you with important fat-soluble nutrients. A whole egg is so nutritious that it should be a part of everyone's diet. Persons who have an abnormally high level of cholesterol in their blood may have to restrict consumption of egg yolk since it is rich in cholesterol. If you are healthy, however, eating whole eggs in a normal, balanced diet will *not* raise your blood cholesterol.

Luckily for humans who eat eggs, nature included lecithin, essential fatty acids, and B vitamins in egg yolk to keep its cholesterol emulsified (softened) for use in the development of a living chick. Cooking an egg tends to destroy lecithin and essential fatty acids, leaving the cholesterol intact. Eggs *must* be cooked, however, to prevent possible poisoning by salmonella, a dangerous form of bacteria. Besides, a raw egg contains avidin, a substance that interferes with absorption of the B vitamin biotin. So while an egg should be cooked before eating it, it should not be overcooked. The trick is to cook the egg just enough to leave the yolk a little soft. Soft-boiled eggs are best. Also, cooking an egg in its shell will conserve nutrients.

HEALTH DRINKS ARE POPULAR

Just about everyone has a formula for a health drink. It's the rare star or celebrity who doesn't mix a special beverage for use as a dietary supplement. High-protein energy drinks are the most popular, especially in Hollywood circles. Practically all of these drinks have the same basic ingredients: powdered protein, brewer's yeast, milk, ice, and flavoring—all mixed in a blender. Fresh fruit or frozen fruit juice concentrate is most often used to flavor a drink. For example, *to make a high-protein milkshake,* you just add a few ice cubes, a couple of tablespoons of powdered protein or powdered nonfat milk, and a banana or a peach (or any fruit of your choice) to a glass of skimmed milk and mix in a blender until the milk is frothy and frosty. *To make an energy drink,* you simply add a little brewer's yeast powder to the high-protein drink and mix with a blender. Yeast is rich in energy-giving B vitamins and other anti-fatigue factors. Until you become

Movie and TV actress *Rosemary Forsythe* suggests that you can do your family a favor by serving them health drinks rather than soda pop and other unwholesome beverages.

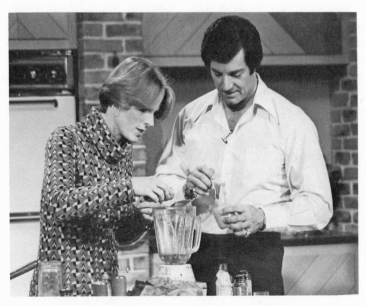

Rosemary Forsythe of "Days of Our Lives," like most Hollywood stars, makes her own special health drink in a blender.

accustomed to the taste of yeast, however, begin with less than a teaspoon of yeast powder per drink and slowly increase the amount to suit your taste.

Here's a simple recipe for an energy drink:

1 quart skimmed milk

½ cup skimmed milk powder

½ cup brewer's yeast powder

1 small can frozen fruit juice concentrate

Mix all these ingredients in a blender and store in a refrigerator for daily use. Each time you drink a glass of the mixture, re-mix the serving with a couple of ice cubes in a blender. To avoid a noisy strain on your blender, you may use crushed ice if you like.

You may, of course, blend almost anything into a health drink, including nuts, yogurt, fruits, vegetables, and oils, depending upon your needs and your taste. Strongly flavored fruit juice concentrate can be used to disguise the taste of liver, yeast, lecithin, and other unappetizing ingredients. With a little imagination and experimentation, you can formulate a health drink that will fit your specific needs—and you can flavor it with your favorite fruit or concentrate.

Physical fitness expert *Jack LaLanne* mixes his own special high-protein energy drink for use as a breakfast beverage. Here is his formula:

6 ounces of unsweetened apple juice

6 ounces low-fat milk

1 ounce 50 percent high-protein powder fortified with vitamins and minerals

2 tablespoons of 80 percent milk-and-egg protein powder

2 tablespoons raw wheat germ

1 tablespoon brewer's yeast powder

3 to 4 large ice cubes

honey as a sweetener if desired

All of these ingredients are mixed in a blender until the ice cubes are adequately crushed.

Jean-Claude Killy, a world champion skier, makes a simple high-protein drink by mixing protein powder, two egg yolks, and a banana into a pint of raw milk. (If you use raw milk, make sure that it's certified.)

At Peter Lupus Leisure Health World, we used a special, balanced breakfast beverage formulated by *Peter Lupus.* Here, revealed for the first time, is the formula for that beverage:

1 large can of frozen orange juice concentrate mixed with 2 cans of water

6 tablespoons of papaya syrup concentrate

1 teaspoon cold-pressed safflower oil

2 tablespoons brewer's yeast powder

1 tablespoon lecithin granules

2 heaping teaspoons soya powder

2 teaspoons low-fat milk powder

2 teaspoons liquid acidophilus

These ingredients are mixed in a blender and kept in a refrigerator. When served, one cupful of the mixture is mixed in a blender with one-third cup of ice.

High-Protein Refresher

If you want a refreshing high-protein drink without the taste of yeast, try this formula:

1 cup skimmed milk

2 tablespoons protein powder

¼ ripe papaya

2 fresh strawberries

chunks of pineapple

1 teaspoon honey

1 raw egg

3 ice cubes

Mix all ingredients in a blender.

There are, of course, many ways to make health drinks without using either protein powder or brewer's yeast. Skimmed milk powder is a tasty source of protein, but some protein powders do not have a pleasant flavor. You have to cultivate a taste for brewer's yeast. So, when you serve friends and guests, you might have to go easy on the use of protein powder and yeast. If you prefer, you can serve blended fruit or vegetable drinks. If you want a *sweet* drink, for example, you can mix fresh fruits with ice and milk in a blender, adding honey as a sweetener if desired—or you may simply serve a mixture of fruit juices. For something that's *not* sweet, a mixture of vegetables can be liquified in a blender, adding vegetable juice and salt as needed.

Former "Miss Canada" *Aniko Farrell* makes a combination drink by mixing apples and carrots. "I have a juicer," she said, "that I use to blend a mixture of apples and carrots. I mix about one-half of each in the juicer and then cool it in a refrigerator." Actress *Dina Merrill* drinks a blended all-vegetable mixture of carrots, celery, beets, and spinach. Actor *Eddie Albert,* who is famous for his health habits and his organic gardening skills, makes an energy drink by blending: three fertile eggs, a half-cup mixture of almonds, pumpkin seeds, and chia seeds; a mixture of cod-liver oil, wheat-germ oil, and soy oil; a cup of fresh grapefruit juice; and a little ginseng root or bee pollen. *Cloris Leachman* and *Billie Jean King* maintain that simple, fresh orange juice is the best energy drink they've found.

There are many formulas for a variety of healthful drinks that can be mixed in a blender. You can alter any formula to suit your taste, but you should always use a blender for best results.

If you cannot resist desserts, follow actress *Heather Menzies'* example and at least eat *wholesome* sweets. You can find many

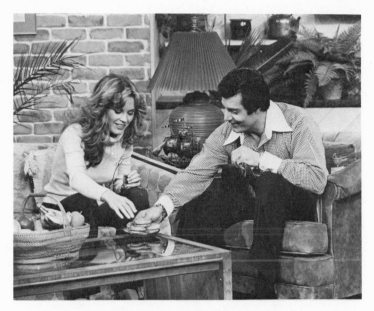

*Heather Menzies, co-star of TV's "Logan's Run," uses all-
natural ingredients when preparing cookies
and other desserts.*

recipes for natural desserts in our book *Doctor Homola's Fat-
Disintegrator Diet* (Parker Publishing Company).

SUMMARY

1. Cooking or preparing foods properly is just as important as selection of foods in building a healthy body.
2. All fruits and vegetables should be eaten raw to assure an adequate supply of fiber and other essential nutrients.
3. With the exception of stir-frying, you should *never* cook with grease or oil.
4. No matter what type of food you're cooking, you should use as little heat, water, and time as possible.
5. Remember that stored foods exposed to air and light lose nutrients.

6. Whenever possible, cook fresh foods each day.

7. Muscular meats should be cooked in the presence of moisture, while fatty meats should be cooked on a rack with *dry* heat.

8. Whole-grain breads and cereals are important sources of fiber, protein, Vitamin E, and B vitamins.

9. Persons on a low-fat diet should use skimmed milk and its products (which must be fermented when there is lactose intolerance).

10. High-protein energy drinks made at home can make a healthful contribution to your diet.

11

Surprising Advice from Health-Conscious Stars and Celebrities

All of the previous chapters of this book are devoted to outlining the *Peter Lupus Body-Improvement Program,* featuring examples of stars and celebrities who follow such a program. In this chapter, we want to present a few in-depth interviews obtained from Hollywood stars who follow their own unique programs. Each of these interviews has something special to offer in helping you help yourself. You'll see that no two programs are exactly alike, even though all of them are apparently beneficial — some in spite of a few bad habits.

After you have read this book and you begin to follow your own program, it's perfectly all right to be original if you follow certain basic guides. For example, if you choose not to eat red meat, you should include milk, cheese, and other animal products to prevent a deficiency in protein, Vitamin B_{12}, and other essential nutrients. If you are underweight, you can eat more of all types of foods, especially those foods that are rich in protein and natural carbohydrate, and you can adopt a form of exercise that enlarges your muscles. If you are overweight, you must select low-calorie foods, supplement your diet with vitamins and minerals, and participate in endurance-type exercise to burn as many calories as possible.

Once you become knowledgeable about foods, supplements, and other factors that play a part in a healthful body-improvement program, you can develop a program that best suits your specific needs. So be sure to read this *entire book* before adopting a program like the one followed by your favorite star or celebrity. If you have any bad habits, you should try to kick them. But don't hesitate to begin a body-improvement program even if you smoke cigarettes or eat candy. You may have to work a little harder to offset a bad habit, but you'll be much healthier and you'll look much better than if you follow no program at all.

Note: All interviews have been placed in alphabetical order.

ED ASNER: NOT A CAPTIVE OF HABITS

The physical features of Ed Asner lend his talent to a great variety of acting roles—from wrestler to newspaper editor. Undoubtedly one of the finest actors in Hollywood, he has earned *five* Emmy Awards for his roles in such television hits as "The Mary Tyler Moore Show," "Rich Man, Poor Man," and "Roots." Presently starring as Lou Grant in the "Lou Grant" series, Ed Asner continues his unbroken string of outstanding performances.

Like all busy actors, Ed Asner must pay close attention to his health habits in order to endure long working hours. Weight control is his biggest problem. Since "The Mary Tyler Moore Show," he has lost 42 pounds! How did he do it? By jogging, fasting, and using liquid protein. Ed hastens to add, however, that he does not recommend liquid protein for everyone. "When I was on the liquid protein diet," he said, "I included fish and chicken and ate a salad at night. I believe I could have skipped the liquid protein and gotten better results.

"I had to quit jogging because of a heel spur. I'm trying to heal the spur because I love running. I don't catch colds when I'm jogging

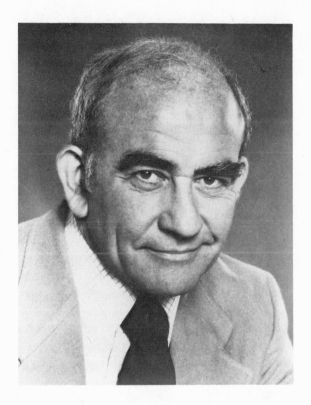

regularly, and my waistline is easier to control. Right now, I'm doing push-ups and sit-ups every day.

"I'm also trying a three-day water fast as opposed to a juice fast. I include coffee and tea but no solid foods. I also take 400 units of Vitamin E, a B complex, and 1,000 milligrams of Vitamin C every day.

"I stopped smoking in November; when I did, my appetite picked up. You know you gain weight even if you don't eat more after you stop smoking. I want to knock the weight off and, for the first time in my life, reach a decent weight while I'm *not* smoking. Then, I *know* I'll feel like a million dollars!

"Normally, I try to include the four basic food groups in my diet— definitely plenty of greens and fresh fruits. I prefer fish and chicken over meats, which I always *broil* when I want to knock off the weight. When I eat out, I never eat in restaurants where the foods are steeped in grease. I never use salt, because I'm well aware that food manufacturers are giving us too much salt already. I read somewhere that we get all the sodium we need in the vegetables we eat. I never use sugar, either. When I cheat and eat ice cream, pastries, or candy, I'm getting sugar, but I never take sugar by itself. For snacks, I prefer *crunchy* objects, such as nuts or popcorn. I *love* mixtures of nuts, raisins, and seeds."

How does Ed Asner fight tension and keep his energy level up? "Food is a great sedative," he answered, "but it's the worst thing in the world for my waistline. The first year of my new show, I was not getting enough sleep, since I had not been able to make the switch over to an hour show very easily. So when I began to drag around on the stage, I'd go more and more to snacks and cigarettes, which, in actuality, were *depriving* me of energy. But it's hard to break old, stupid habits. I now know that I can *never* use fatigue as an excuse for eating.

"There's a book out called *Relaxation Response,* which is an American lay version of transcendental meditation. The last chapter of the book tells you to disassociate yourself from the aggravating factors and to use a process of slowly *counting* away your tension. I've used this procedure a couple of times and it has taken me down.

"To keep my energy up, I try to get adequate sleep at night. I get my feet off the ground during the day whenever I can. I do that even when I'm not tired. If I have 15 minutes with no pressing duties, I lie down and shut my eyes. The recuperative and restorative value of only a minute of such a procedure is enormous.

"I can never sleep more than six hours, but I like the luxury of staying in bed seven hours. It's getting more difficult to sleep in my later years because my sleep is more easily interrupted by noise.

"Alcohol relaxes me. I usually drink a vodka or Scotch on the rocks, but I limit the use of alcohol. There was a time when I overindulged, but not anymore. I find that I can better gauge my limits with straight liquor than with mixed drinks. When I have mixed drinks, I usually discover the worm in the apple too late. I often go for a week or two without having a drink. When I do drink, I just get a buzz on and then stop.

"Training yourself to do without is probably the healthiest thing in the world. If you are a smoker, for example, you should try doing without cigarettes for one day just to show yourself that you can do it. My dad was an orthodox Jew. From Friday sundown to Saturday sundown, all his life, he refrained from smoking. I think it would be wonderful for everyone to *prove* to themselves that they are not a captive of anything, be it booze, cigarettes, or food."

Like Ed Asner, you should be the master of your habits so that you can protect yourself from harmful extremes. Even in the performance of healthful exercise and good eating habits, it's possible to become a captive of extremes. Persons who feel compelled to maintain the ability to jog several miles daily, for example, may be as much a captive as a smoker or a drinker. So remember that the judgment needed to maintain good health must be tempered with wisdom and good sense.

JOHN BERADINO: FROM PROFESSIONAL BALL PLAYER TO MOVIE ACTOR

What's the longest running, most popular daytime show on television? You guessed it—ABC's "General Hospital," a soap that commands as much attention as the sunrise. Its star, John Beradino, who portrays Chief-of-Staff Dr. Steve Hardy, has been with the show since its beginning in 1963! John first started acting at the age of seven as a member of "Our Gang" in the movies. He became a professional baseball player in 1939 and was playing second base for the Cleveland Indians when they won the World Series in 1948. John resumed his movie and television career in 1953 after suffering a leg injury.

How does a busy actor who was once a professional ball player keep in shape? "I play tennis," says John. "Some of the people here use a Pacer Mat on the set to jump up and down and jog on to keep their blood circulating. But my exercising has always been in a competitive vein. I've never been one for jogging or exercising alone. I like to bowl or play tennis so that I can *compete* against someone.

"I had the cartilage in my left knee removed over a year ago and it still isn't up to par. So I can't do as much as I want to do.

"I've never really had a weight problem. I just eat what I've always eaten. I don't think I've picked up more than five or six pounds since I've quit playing ball. I eat the basic staples and cut out fat as much as possible. I don't live a Hollywood life, so I go home each night and eat my wife's home-cooked meals. She might have a roast with potatoes

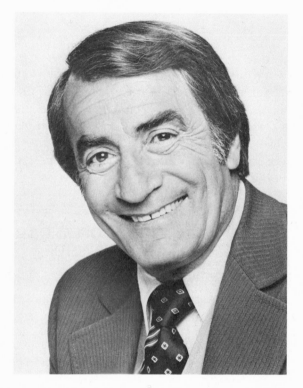

and string beans, for example. I like tuna, chicken, and fish. I snack on fruits.

"I'm very constant in the type of foods I eat. I really don't experiment with foods. Even when I go to an Italian restaurant, I'll probably have shrimp scampi with garlic; that's one of my favorites. When I find something I like, I stick with it. It's either the scampi or some fish with a little pasta on the side. I'm not a dessert man, so I don't eat desserts often."

The most relaxing part of John's day is coming home each night to his wife, Marjorie, and their two young children, Katherine Anne and John Anthony. "Just being with them relaxes me and relieves my tension," John says. "I'm really a home person. This is one of the reasons why I prefer being on a daytime show. I like to go home every night.

"I've always been an eight-hour man when it comes to sleep. If I don't get my eight hours, I'm in trouble. I go to bed early and I like to arise early. I like to see and feel the morning—going outside and smelling everything. The more daylight you see, the more you enjoy life."

Early to bed and early to rise is a good procedure for all of us to follow in improving our health. Make sure that *you* get adequate sleep. Enhance your health and your life by being a "home person" as much as possible.

SUSAN BROWN: HEALTH ADVICE
FROM A TELEVISION DOCTOR

Susan Brown has had numerous roles in a variety of movie and television films ranging from "Andromeda Strain" to "Barney Miller." But she is probably best known for her role as Dr. Gail Adamson on "General Hospital," the longest running daytime television show ever produced in Hollywood. Susan's roles in "Dr. Kildare," "Marcus Welby," "Doc Elliot," and now "General Hospital" make it difficult to believe that she is not a nurse or a doctor. So it seems quite natural to ask her about health care. Some of Susan's fans refuse to believe that she is *not* a doctor! In any event, here's what she had to say about exercise and other aspects of personal health care.

"I've taken dance classes through the years, and I play tennis. I think yoga is wonderful. I have a pool at home where I swim. I find that it's hard to make myself jog and do things like that. But when the Pacer Mat came along, I thought it was *terrific*. It's like a little trampoline that you can run on or bounce on. I put it in front of my television set and use it while I'm watching the news or whatever—and 15 or 20 minutes go by very quickly. This way, I'm entertained while I'm exercising. I use the Pacer Mat every day now, and it's the only exercise I'm doing consistently. It's not as hard on your feet and knees as when running on pavement.

"I've never had to diet. If I do gain a few pounds, I would rather eliminate a meal or two than do without something I like to eat during a meal. Then, when I do eat, I eat what I want. I'm not a vegetarian. I don't eat desserts and I exercise regularly, so I don't often gain enough

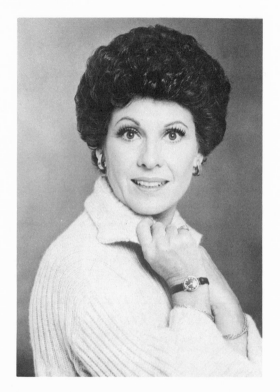

weight to force me to eliminate a meal. My calorie intake pretty well balances my calorie output.

"I have always believed in taking vitamins. I take 800 units of Vitamin E with my orange juice each morning. I take two to three alfalfa tablets each day so that I won't develop arthritis. I also take a B complex and about 500 milligrams of Vitamin C every day.

"I shampoo my hair three or four times a week with a pH balance protein shampoo, and I use a conditioner. I'm really most careful about my face. I try not to get my face out in the sun too much. I've found a *wonderful* thing for eyelashes. Rubbing *castor oil* on eyelashes with a Q-tip revitalizes lashes and makes them grow! It's better than any eyelash cream I've ever heard of. It takes about three months to grow an eyelash, so you don't want to lose too many, especially if you damage them by wearing false eyelashes.

"Crisco is as good as anything to rub on nails, since it's made from vegetable oil. A dermatologist told me that one of the best things you can use on dry skin is Crisco. You can rub it on cuticles, on dry hands, on your legs, your elbows, or anything that's dry."

Susan Brown may only be a make-believe doctor, but three years as Dr. Adamson on "General Hospital," combined with her personal example, certainly lends credibility to her health advice. A good physical appearance enhanced by good health can lend credibility to you, too, in everything you do in life!

JOSEPH CAMPANELLA:
"MY FAMILY KEEPS ME YOUNG"

Versatile Joe Campanella, whose voice is as well known as his face, didn't tell us exactly how old he is—only that he is "over 50." We do know, however, that he looks and acts 10 years younger than he

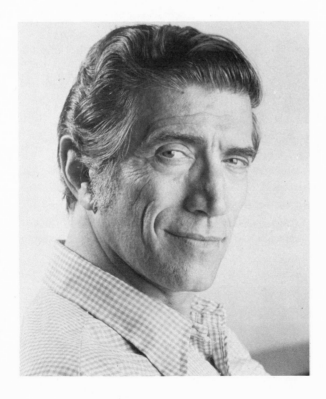

really is. "I have six boys ranging in age from one to thirteen," Joe began. "I have a young family, and I think that helps keep me young. I participate in sports with my boys, and I manage and coach them in baseball, basketball, and other athletic activities. I'm needed by my family; I'm necessary. I want to be a part of this as long as I can. I want to enjoy my family and see them through high school. I want to see them start out their lives, and the only way I can do that is by staying in shape. I'm six feet two inches tall and weigh 185 pounds. I still wear shirts my mother made for me when I was 16 years old! I still have a 33-inch waistline. So I'm staying about the same. It's important not to succumb to the *suggestion* of old age. You can stay young in attitude if not in years."

We agree with Joe that there isn't a better reason for staying in shape than to lengthen your life so that you can enjoy your family. Even if you aren't particularly interested in the body beautiful, remember that the good health and longevity that come from taking good care of yourself will add to your *enjoyment* of life. If you love your family and they need you, you owe it to yourself *and* your family to preserve your health. Take a clue from Joe Campanella and use your family for motivation in your body-improvement program. Your family life will, in turn, provide you with plenty of incentive for living.

"I don't have one conditioning program," Joe continued. "Once every three or four years, I'll get real enthusiastic and go into a gym and really get into shape. But I never stop exercising. I go through calisthenic routines at home—and I use a Bullworker. If I get bored with one routine, I'll go to another.

"They say that the worst exercise is housework—and it is unless you use it right. You can exercise your legs by going up and down the stairs a lot. When I lift something, I lift it properly, but I may lift it several times for exercise. When I lift my young son, I'll press him over my head a few times. He loves it and I'm getting exercise at the same time. When I reach for a top shelf, I'll stretch rather than stand on a chair. I wish I had the discipline to follow a definite program, but I don't. So I do something around the house every day.

"I've always been slightly underweight. As a matter of fact, I've always had to eat to keep my weight up. And in order for me to eat enough to do this, I have to exercise to stimulate my appetite. So I have a healthy chain going. I don't have trouble with cholesterol or anything. I eat the foods I like to eat, but I eat in moderation. I like to snack on Italian cheeses, sometimes a bowl of cold cereal, such as granola. We eat fresh fruit every night. There is *always* fresh fruit in the house—whatever is in season.

"Another thing that helps me in my discipline is drinking a lot of water. I try to keep my system flushed. Everytime I pass a sink, I'll drink half a glass of water—not a full glass but a *half* a glass. I drink a total of eight to 10 glasses of water a day.

"The one weakness I have is for pasta and bread. But because of my weight I can afford to eat them. I *burn* them off. I use a lot of energy walking. When I take my car to the garage, for example, I never ask for a ride back; I *walk* back. I often ride a bicycle to the store.

"I take a good, general, all-around vitamin-and-mineral supplement. I take protein tablets with me when I travel. I also take wheat germ oil and Vitamin E. Taking them makes me feel good. All of my boys take multiple vitamins and minerals. The last time I took my four oldest boys to the dentist, they went in to have their teeth cleaned and not one of them had a cavity. It's not the toothpaste they're using, it's the food they eat and the supplements they take!

"When I come home tired and tense at the end of a long day, just walking into the house rejuvenates me. There's so much activity going on, so many problems to take care of, that the sudden change from the studio to my home brings me back into the real world and I begin to relax. Then, when I hit the bed at night, I go right to sleep.

"I stopped using aftershave lotions. I now use Vitamin A-and-D cream on my face after I shave. This helps my skin. I believe that Vitamin E and wheat germ oil also help. I wash my hair every other day. I've never believed in the everyday shampoo because it makes my hair dry and unmanageable.

"My advice to anyone who want to stay in shape is to *do what you can to stay active.* Walk more. Ride a bicycle. I run some, but I hate jogging. What I do is alternately sprint and walk. You can get adequate exercise simply by going up and down stairs. You should always walk instead of riding when you have a choice. The important thing is to do something that *you* can do and then do it *regularly.*"

According to Joe Campanella, there isn't any reason why any reasonably healthy person cannot get adequate exercise around the house. So the old excuse "I don't have time to exercise" is not valid for most of us. Enough said!

JAMES FARENTINO AND MICHELE LEE: CAREER, FAMILY, AND GOOD HEALTH!

James Farentino and Michele Lee were married in 1966 and now have a son, David Michael. Both James and Michele have a long, long list of movie, television, and stage credits. Michele has even recorded a hit album for Columbia Records! With James co-starring in the forthcoming movie "Last Countdown" with Suzanne Somers and Kirk Douglas, and Michele co-starring with Don Murray in a new television series called "Knots Landing," both Frank and Michele enjoy a successful career as well as a happy marriage. Their example demonstrates that it's possible to have it all: a successful career, a happy marriage, a close family, and good health. Best of all, their son, David, is getting off to a good start with good health habits, which is most important early in life.

"David is very interested in physical fitness," Michele said proudly, "and he's particular about what he eats. I firmly believe that your eating habits are formed when you're young. If a parent restricts sweet intake, or allows sweets in certain forms, an *apple* can become a dessert. David won't eat fat, and he hates salt. It's the psychology behind how you *label* foods that molds eating habits. My son is very sophisticated in his eating habits. We even allow him in the kitchen to help cook. He makes a *good* salad."

Most of us eat three meals a day. Some of us eat only when we're hungry. James Farentino has found that eating only *one meal* a day is best for him. "But I eat a very *healthy* meal," James explained, "and I don't snack or eat sweets. I really don't have a desire to snack, and I just do not like sweets. I have been *conditioned* to eat this way. I eat a lot of vegetables. Chicken is one of my favorites. I cook chicken all the time. It's a dish you can prepare 150 different ways. The one big vice I have in terms of eating is pasta."

Michele Lee eats *two* meals a day—lunch and dinner. She has only coffee in the morning. "I sometimes have a tuna fish sandwich with avocado on egg bread," she said. "I *love* salads. I put *everything*

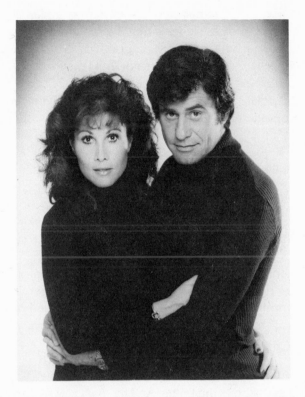

in my salads—sunflower seeds, or nuts, crepes, raisins, cheese, tomatoes, fresh cauliflower or broccoli, and so on. Since my husband has been taking over the cooking chores, he has been making me *fat* by cooking too much pasta! I want to get back into Chinese cooking—with a lot of chicken and stir-fried vegetables. We try to stay away from red meats, and we don't add salt to our foods.

"I gave up smoking about four years ago to improve my health. When I quit smoking I found it more difficult to control my weight, but I'll *never* go back to smoking."

Michele gets her exercise by dancing and by pedaling a stationary bicycle in her house. "I pedal my bike every day," Michele said, "and I set the tension on the bike so that my heart rate reaches 130 to 150 beats per minute—for at least 20 minutes—for cardiovascular exercise. I'm very conscious about cardiovascular exercise now because of all the talk about heart disease."

James plays racquetball and works out on a Nautilus exercise machine in a health club. He feels that the resistive exercise provided by a Nautilus machine also has a good cardiovascular effect. "I normally only play racquetball," he said, "but I plan to work out on the Nautilus three times a week—every other day—for three months to stretch the muscles I don't use in racquetball. During that time, I'll play racquetball on alternate days and take the weekends off. After three months, I'll go back to racquetball five days a week."

One final question for Michele: What do you do for your skin and hair? "With my hair as long as it is now," she replied, "I have to wash it at least every other day, and I always use a conditioning cream. I use a water base make-up on my skin. I prefer to keep my skin as free of grease as I can. I use plain soap and water to clean my skin, but I use a *mild* soap. I try to avoid overexposure to the sun, since sun ages the skin."

James and Michele offer this general advice to persons who are seeking better health: "Don't smoke, do some sort of aerobic exercise, such as swimming, and stretch all the muscles of the body in some other forms of exercise. Eat as well as possible, have a couple of drinks a day, make love, and laugh a lot."

If you have children, remember that the sooner you begin to mold their health habits the better. And the best way to do this is to set a good example for them to follow.

HEALTHY LIVING IS A WAY OF LIFE FOR TED KNIGHT

Super healthy Ted Knight has been following a disciplined health regimen for 30 years, and it has paid off for him *and* his family. "We've *always* been interested in good health and proper eating habits for ourselves and our children," Ted explained, "and the living proof of that is what our kids look like. We have three kids—all *giants*. We *all* are involved in good eating habits.

"My wife, Dorothy, is the one who started us on our health regimens. She got me involved in the Price-Pottenger Nutrition Foundation, which has proved beyond a shadow of any doubt that

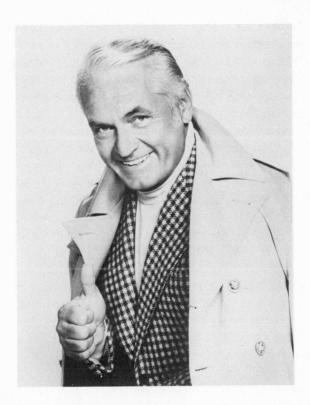

western civilized processed food is not only debilitating and deleterious but also creates dental problems that do not occur when you eat only natural foods.

"I'm not a fanatic, but I'm very careful about the foods I take in. I eat fresh fruits and vegetables. I don't eat packaged meats or canned goods. I minimize my meat intake. I eat beef only if it has not been contaminated by additives or hormones. I eat mostly poultry and fish. I *never* charbroil my meats.

"My diet is basically very simple. There are an infinite variety of simple ways to prepare fruits and vegetables. I usually eat my vegetables raw or steamed, with as little cooking as possible. The more raw the food, the more nutritious it is. If you boil out your food, you might as well chew on paper.

"I'm very selective when I eat out, but it's never as good as when I eat at home. So I always take double doses of supplemental vitamins with me. I avoid sauces and things of that nature, and I make certain that the salads are cleansed properly. I even check the kitchen! I want to know who the cooks are and how they prepare the food before I eat it. I try to avoid restaurants as much as I can. I don't eat fried stuff at all. I'll seek out vegetables on my plate more than I will the main course and then cut my supply in half.

"I don't have to go on a special diet to control my body weight. I may have dropped 10 or 12 pounds over the past few years, but all I do is watch what I put into my system. I don't eat processed foods or desserts. I never use sugar—only honey. I've found that since I've stayed away from sweets I can't really stand anything sweet anymore. Sweets have become sickening to me. What happens is that your palate becomes more sensitive to sweets. An orange or an apple can be tremendously sweet. A handful of dates is more than enough to keep me satisfied.

My only weakness now is a couple of cups of coffee a day, but I never put sugar in it. Drinking coffee is the *only* thing I do that is not good for me. I occasionally have a glass of wine when I'm relaxing with friends, but that's as bad as I get. I've never smoked, and I won't stay in a room where people are smoking.

"I supplement my food with vitamins. I average three or four grams of Vitamin C a day, for example. I take it in various forms throughout the day. I take it in capsule form and as ascorbic powder. I take it with me in packets when I travel. When I feel a cold coming on, I *double* the dosage. The result is I never catch a cold. I never have a problem, even when people around me are hacking and sneezing."

Like all successful actors, Ted Knight has a busy and exhausting schedule and must constantly battle tension and fatigue. "I sometimes have to get up at six o'clock in the morning," he said, "and I don't get home until after the sun goes down. When I feel that I need to relax at night before I go to bed, I'll take a combination of Vitamin C, magnesium, and B complex together, which acts as a tranquilizer because it feeds the nerves. It supplements something that you burned out in your body that needs to be replaced. I *never* take valium and other tranquilizing drugs. I prefer to put in an hour a day of some kind of exercise, which relaxes me.

"I alternate methods of exercise. Doing the same thing all the time can be boring and tedious. Right now, I'm thinking about buying an exercising cycle. Sometimes I jog, walk, or do wind sprints, depending upon how I feel. I just go the limits of what feels good to me on that particular day. I don't have a regimen where I determine beforehand to do five or six miles a day. I don't think that's necessary—as long as you do enough to keep yourself toned. I do some kind of exercise *every day*—anything to fill in an hour. I try to do at least 20 minutes at 75 percent effort to get my pulse rate up to 120 beats per minute. I make sure that my heart is beating fast and I'm breathing deeply.

"If you live in an area where you're allergic to the pollen in the air, find a bee hive in that area and collect some honey from that hive. You can immunize yourself by eating honey made from the flowers that bother you. It's like taking a shot of serum."

Ted Knight has a beautiful head of hair. Does he do anything special for his hair? "I used to watch my mother put her head down between her knees and brush her hair 100 strokes," he answered. "I do that everyday, but not with a brush. After I get through exercising and blood is circulating through my system, I'll comb my hair and massage my scalp. I do that *every day.* I don't know whether it makes any difference or not because I have a brother with identical hair who doesn't do it at all. I'm healthier than my brother, however, and I know it's because of the difference in the way we take care of ourselves.

"My brother and I had similar body chemistry when we were growing up. He's a year and a half older than I am. But he hasn't had the advantage of acquiring vanities—and I mean that in a positive sense. I think it's good to be vain, because to look your best you have to think a lot of yourself. You have to do that to stay in this business. My brother never had that. So he just lived a kind of slothful, day-to-day mundane life. His doctors have told him that they want to replace his knee joints. He's arthritic, he has gout, he's had a mild heart seizure, he's 40 pounds overweight, and he looks 20 years older and acts 30 years older than I am!

"Now, I, on the other hand, for 30 years, have been keeping myself as fit as possible to look good for the cameras. In the past five or six years, I've intensified my awareness of what my machinery is all about, and I'm taking care of it more and more. So I feel as healthy now as I did 30 years ago. My brother, on the other hand, is falling apart. I don't mean to demean him in any way. It's just a fact of life. He didn't take care of himself. I'm in good condition because of the vair aspects of my business; it *forced* me to take care of myself.

"When people are determined to stay on a crash course of self destruction, you can't tell them anything. I've talked to some people until I'm blue in the face, but to no avail. People who are determined to make themselves better are going to find a way, regardless of what you and I say. They'll look to you if they're really interested, and they'll seek out the information they need. If they look for a means to improve their condition, they'll find it."

Thanks, Ted. We hope that readers who want to improve their health will seek out this book and find the information they need.

THE MODERATE APPROACH
OF PETER LAWFORD

Most of us have to work hard at keeping a lean body with good skin and a healthy head of hair. Some people, however, are blessed with outstanding physical qualities that are natural and easy to maintain. These lucky people don't have to worry about losing hair or staying on a strict diet. All they have to do is maintain their health with general measures that do not require sacrifice or a disciplined regimen. Veteran actor Peter Lawford is one of these lucky people. Over the years as a successful actor in movies, on television, and on the stage, Peter has consistently weighed about 160 pounds. Except for graying hair, he has changed very little physically at a time in life when the average person is literally falling apart. What is his secret? Probably a way of life that he developed at a very early age.

"I've been athletically inclined all my life," Peter explained, "and it has borne me good stead. I started out playing tennis when I was seven. When I came to America, I went into surfing, which is an incredible way to stay in shape. My physical condition is really the result of a combination of things. I used to pump iron or lift weights. I was never a Muscle Beach person, but I was always in good shape. I played tennis and surfed and then got into golf. Now I'm back to tennis again.

"The mistake a lot of people make is that they're athletic in school and college, and, unless they go on to professional athletics,

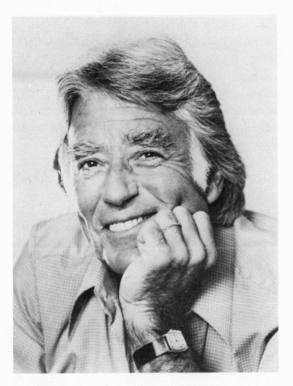

they end up behind a desk. Then, after 20 years of sitting behind a desk, they suddenly start jogging, expecting to get back into shape overnight. It's important to *continue* some kind of physical activity that's not boring—something that does not become a monkey on your back.

"I'm not a jogger. I enjoy walking, but I set a pace. Someone told me a long time ago—and it makes sense to me—that if you get out of breath, really out of breath, at least once a day, your heart will stay strong and your arteries won't harden.

"There are, of course, a lot of things I do that are not good for me. Admittedly, I smoke, which, according to the Surgeon General, is a bad trip. Once I stopped smoking for 18 months and then went back to it. But I don't smoke as much as I used to. I light one and then I'll put it away.

"As far as my body weight goes, I'm really a very lucky person. I can eat pasta seven nights a week without gaining weight. I don't have a weight problem, and I'm still pretty firm. The thing is, I'm not a big eater—which is something I can't take credit for. You know the old trick of pushing the plate away. I don't have to do that. I take small portions because I just don't eat much. But sometimes I go on an ice cream binge. I guess that's my monkey. My metabolism seems to take care of it, however.

"I get my vitamins in health drinks, which I love. Sometimes I make my drinks with orange juice and milk. I add protein powder, a couple of eggs, a banana, or sometimes a few strawberries for a different taste. To me, a health drink is a great way to get going in the morning. Sometimes I have the drink for lunch—whenever I feel like it. Sometimes I add brewer's yeast. I use a soya protein powder that has *everything* in it—all the vitamins and minerals. I take extra Vitamin C when I have a cold, and I get some extra sleep.

"Normally, six to seven hours of sleep are enough for me. If I sleep 10 hours, I get loggy. I can refresh my body by taking naps. I can sleep on a plane or in a corner standing up. I feel sorry for people who can't take cat naps."

Peter Lawford doesn't take credit for his luxurious head of hair. "I don't do anything special for my skin and hair," he admitted. "I wash my hair once a day with a protein shampoo that contains a conditioner. And that's it. I'm not a health nut. I just try to take care of myself. Some people have to work at it; I feel sorry for them.

"I don't follow any special rules in selecting my foods. I'm not a big meat eater. I love fish, and I'm crazy about lamb chops. But I'm not one of those people who wants a steak every day. I love liver and fresh vegetables. I cook my vegetables by steaming them a little. When I eat out, I usually order something I'm familiar with, such as scrambled eggs. I don't like rich food, such as sauces and so on.

"I snack on yogurt. I don't like *plain* yogurt, however. I like it with fruit, such as bananas or blueberries. But the plain yogurt, I can't have it."

Peter believes that staying healthy and fit is largely mental. "I've seen people stay on a strict diet and have the worst-looking skin with their hair falling out. There is obviously something else wrong with their body. Mental attitude may be a factor. When eating for better health, the simpler the diet the better. I'm a very plain kind of eater. This may be one reason why I don't gain weight. If I ate like a lot of people, I probably would gain weight.

"Depression or a bad mood is probably caused more by mental attitude than by bad food. You can get out of depression if you're lucky enough to have a natural kind of stamina, which I seem to have."

Much of Peter Lawford's "natural stamina" can undoubtedly be attributed to his preference for "plain foods," his life-long use of recreational exercise, and his daily use of a multiple vitamin-and-mineral fortified high-protein drink. So even if you are blessed with good physical qualities, you should do as Peter does and preserve these qualities by at least taking moderately good care of yourself. It'll pay off in the long run.

PAUL LYNDE'S BATTLE
AGAINST OVERWEIGHT

Paul Lynde is one of America's funniest comedians. He was voted the "Funniest Man of the Year" by the American Academy of Humor in 1975, and in 1976 the American Guild of Variety Artists selected him as the "Comedian of the Year." But when it comes to diet and weight, Paul is dead serious. Controlling his body weight has always been a problem for him—and the problem started when he gained 100 pounds at the age of 10 while recovering from an appendectomy. At one time, Paul weighed as much as 260 pounds! But not today. Although he manages to keep his weight down, it's still a struggle for him. He weighs 190 pounds at the present time but prefers to weigh about 170 pounds dressed.

"I've been on every diet known to man," Paul confessed, "and I succeeded on all of them, but the weight always comes back. Someone should write a book on how to keep the weight off when you lose it. Most of the people I know have dieted all their life, and it has been up and down for them—like a yoyo.

"My midwestern background in the potato salad belt has a lot to do with my eating habits. My mother died never using our broiler. Salad was always potato salad or Waldorf. We *never* had a green salad. If anything was green, she'd cream it! When you eat that way for many years, those are your taste buds for life. I would like *gravy* as a beverage.

"I like sandwiches; they're easy—no mess and you don't need

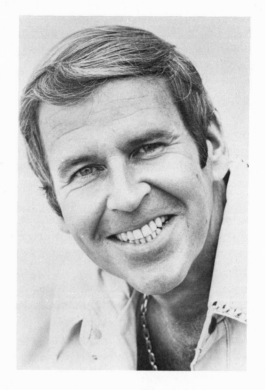

silverware. But I like Miracle Whip on my sandwiches. I *love* Miracle Whip! It's hard to change my taste buds, so I have to keep going on diets. And it's the biggest bore in the world because I would rather eat than anything.

"When I'm on the road, I try to limit my diet to a broiled piece of meat or seafood with a big salad. But I'm never hungry before giving a performance. So I usually eat *after* a performance. Unfortunately, it's usually so late when I get out of the theater that there aren't any good restaurants open. If someone stays open for you and they know you're coming, they want you to eat the specialty of the house, which is usually fattening.

"One of the biggest regrets of my life is that I didn't get into exercise as a teenager. I took choir instead of gym, because if you took choir you didn't have to take gym. I'd do *anything* to avoid exercise. I played bass drum in the band, which got me out of gym, too. Probably one of the major disappointments in my life is that my family did not encourage me in sports and athletics. If you wait until you're 50 years old to begin exercising, it's hard. The only exercise I get now is going from bed to chair!

"Alcohol is an enormous problem for me; it's so fattening. I use it as a shield when I go to parties because you're involved with *lots* of boring people. So you fortify yourself. I'm strictly a social drinker. I would *never* think of having a drink at home alone. It's not even on my mind. It's just built-in conditioning to drink socially for fortification. I've always felt that the only way I could ever solve my weight problem or quit drinking is to get out of show business so that I can live without those pressures. Alcohol relaxes me, but I know it's bad for my body.

"Having a good body is important. I think the most guarded secret is what you think you look like nude. This results in many inhibitions. If I had a gorgeous body, I'd be nude all the time. A beautiful body is a beautiful thing to see, and it provides incentive to stay in shape rather than wear robes all the time. I think most people are ashamed of their bodies, so they hide in robes. I say if you've got it flaunt it! I wear *my* robe when I take a shower."

We agree, Paul, that a beautiful body is a beautiful thing to see. And a beautiful body is usually a *healthy* body. If you study our dietary recommendations (outlined in Chapter 1), your problems will be solved, and you can shed those robes forever!

HOW GAVIN MACLEOD LOST
MORE THAN 80 POUNDS OF FAT

Gavin MacLeod is a hard-working actor who has more than 300 movie, television, and stage credits to his name, including two years in the "McHale's Navy" television series and seven years as a co-star on "The Mary Tyler Moore Show." He has been nominated *twice* for the "Golden Globe" award as the best supporting actor in a comedy series. He is presently starring in the ABC-TV series "The Love Boat."

In his role as Captain Merrill Stubing, Gavin MacLeod is a familiar figure to television viewers. Yet, many people do not associate him with his hundreds of past movie and television performances. Why?

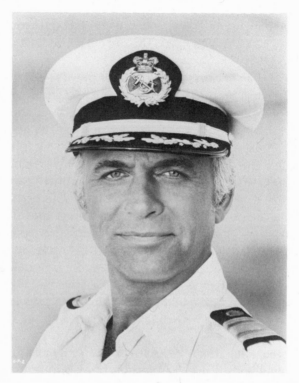

Because many people do not recognize the new Gavin MacLeod! At 47 years of age, he looks so much better today than he did in years past that he does not even look like the same person. When Gavin co-starred in "McHale's Navy" in the role of Happy Haines 17 years ago, he weighed 265 pounds! Today, as Captain Stubing in the "Love Boat" series, he weighs 184 pounds and looks completely transformed. In fact, he now looks so much better overall that it's difficult to believe that the Happy Haines of 1962 is the Captain Stubing of 1979. How did he make such miraculous changes in his physical appearance?

We made a special effort to interview Gavin MacLeod. We wanted to learn first-hand the health secrets of this Hollywood star who seems to be growing younger rather than older. We found that part of his secret is his wife, Patti, whom he met in 1972. Under her influence, he quit smoking and drinking and became a vegetarian. "Patti gets me going," Gavin admits. "She is the impetus for the way I look and think today. She has introduced me to all the positive thoughts of life."

With a new mental attitude and a positive outlook, Gavin combines mental and physical factors to make the most of his time and talents. His high energy level and his enthusiasm for his work add up to *happy* work days that are as productive as they are therapeutic.

"The character I'm playing and my approach to life keep me enthusiastic about my work," Gavin explained. "If I have a groovy scene to do—a scene I've been working on—I can't wait to get to the studio to do it . . . . I work on a high energy level. That, I think, comes from my enthusiasm for life."

To maintain the source of his energy and to control his body weight, Gavin eliminates red meats from his diet and includes eggs, fish, and other animal products in a vegetarian-type diet. Here's how he described his diet: "In the morning, I will have a banana or a hard-boiled egg. For lunch, I'll have a lettuce-and-tomato salad with a tablespoon of oil and vinegar. The salad is not very big—just enough to fill my stomach. In the afternoon, I'll have either an apple, an orange, a peach—some kind of fruit. Dinner, which is my big meal, starts with a salad. This is a *large* salad consisting mainly of romaine lettuce. We have that with tomatoes. We also have sunflower seeds, cucumbers, and parsley with an herb dressing—a sizeable salad. We wait 15 minutes before eating something else. Then we will have a steamed vegetable, usually zucchini, which is God's food. Maybe we'll have a piece of fish or a piece of chicken—not necessarily. Sometimes we have a baked potato, which will take the place of the chicken or the fish. We don't use salt.

"Patti makes health drinks in a blender, using real papaya and other fruits. I enjoy a coconut-pineapple drink.

"I fast one day a week. During the fast, I drink only distilled water or I have zucchini soup at the end of the day.

"Obviously, I have a very controlled diet. I'm the kind of guy who lives by habit. I have to discipline myself or I go right to pieces.

"My only weakness is desserts. I *love* desserts. When I stopped drinking, I went to desserts because of the natural sugar. That's my poison—starch. If I had only two or three more years to live, I'd live on starch alone to satisfy my craving.

"I don't take any vitamins or minerals or anything—nothing for the last eight years. My doctor says that if you eat the right combination of foods you don't need to take anything. I'm not against taking vitamins. Maybe someday I will. All I can say is that the way I eat now is working good for me."

For exercise, Gavin rides a bicycle and practices yoga (including standing on his head for five minutes). Every morning when he showers, he contracts his abdominal muscles isometrically and then pounds them 50 times with both hands.

What's the secret of self improvement? "You have to like yourself to improve yourself," Gavin says. "Find things in yourself that *you* like and start working on those things to make yourself *love* yourself. When you like yourself, you start doing good things for yourself. You're an important person—a special person. When you think that way about yourself, you *have* to do good for yourself."

We think that's good advice for readers who want to follow a body-improvement program. Start liking yourself *now.*

ROBERT PINE AND GWYNNE GILFORD: A TEAM ALL THE WAY TO THE TOP

Robert Pine and Gwynne Gilford are husband and wife. Both star in their own television series—Robert in "CHiPs" and Gwynne in "A New Kind of Family." But at home they are a team, each helping the other to grow and improve their health. "Since we're both actors," Gwynne says, "We really help one another because we understand each other's needs."

As a former medical student, Robert keeps a scientific watch on his family's health habits. "I have just started taking vitamins recently," he admitted. "I have never been a big vitamin taker. There is so much that's not known about vitamins from a scientific point of view. There is now a lot of talk about Vitamin C and what it does for you. Norman Cousins recently published his story in *Saturday Review* about how he cured himself of a crippling disease by taking large doses of Vitamin C. When heavyweights like Cousins and Dr. Linus Pauling start saying that taking Vitamin C can be beneficial, the medical community takes notice. I think that in the coming years, when these things are proved, there'll be an upsurge in the use of vitamins. I now take a vitamin packet, which I carry with me, that contains *all* the important vitamins."

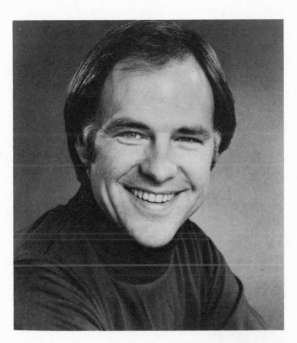

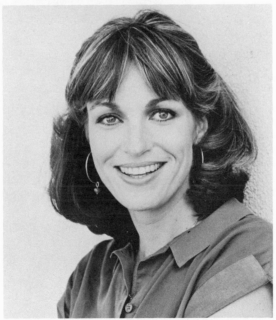

Gwynne confessed that she does not yet take vitamin supplements. "Other than Vitamin C, which I take and give to my daughter, I don't really take supplements," she said. "I'm going to wait and see how Robert does on vitamins. If he improves dramatically, I'll start taking them."

Both Robert and Gwynne get plenty of exercise. "I used to jog three or four miles a day," Robert said, "but I have bad knees and they started to cause problems. So I save my knees for tennis and racquetball. When I go to the gym, I do special exercises to strengthen my knees and legs. I try to swim about four times a week. I do 70 push-ups and about 40 sit-ups every day, at least six days a week. I don't always do the same amount of exercise every day, depending upon my schedule and how I feel, but I always do *something*. I never compete with myself, because if you force yourself to do too much you'll eventually give up. When I am unable to exercise for a while, I'll take a step back. When I'm exercising regularly, however, I at least try not to do less than I did the day before. Then, when I feel like it, I'll do a little extra exercise."

Gwynne gets her exercise by dancing and playing racquetball. "I *love* racquetball!" she exclaimed. "I also like tennis. I've been dancing since I was two years old. I took ballet for 12 years. Jazz is what I'm doing now, because I enjoy it and it makes me feel good and look good. Because we're in such a visible business, we *have* to look good. So we're geared to exercise. It's a way of life for me. I have always exercised, and I'm going to keep on exercising. You can train your mind to look forward to exercising, so that it becomes the treat of the day.

"We're both aware of our diets all the time," Gwynne continued. "So we eat very simple meals. We eat a lot of vegetables, and they're always steamed. We use a steamer to preserve nutrients as much as possible. Our daughter *loves* vegetables cooked this way. Of course, we also eat some vegetables raw. We don't eat a lot of meat. We prefer fish and chicken. And we like brown rice. We really have simple meals. We try to avoid animal fat as much as possible. We do not use salt on our foods. We try to cut all the sugar out of our diet, too, but it's difficult. Our biggest weakness is ice cream. We recently switched to frozen yogurt, which is better. We don't keep sweets in the house. We prefer to snack on fruit, such as apples."

"Instead of giving our daughter soft drinks," Robert injected, "we give her a 'fizz drink' made by mixing equal amounts of grape juice and Perrier water. Katie is only six years old, but she is already aware of good health habits."

Like many of us, Robert and Gwynne have found that an occasional drink at the end of a long, tense day is a great tranquilizer. "It forces you to slow down if you don't have a natural way to do it," Robert explained. "But I certainly believe that the *natural* way is far superior to something chemical like alcohol. We do occasionally have a glass or two of wine with our meals, however."

Gwynne finds companionship great for relieving tension. "After coming home from a hard day," she said, "I think that what we have going for us as actors is that we can go through certain mental exercises to help each other." Robert voiced his agreement. "I think that's important," he said. "A lot of people don't talk. They come home and watch television or something. I think one of the reasons to be married is to have someone to listen to you so that you can talk out your frustrations and decelerate by letting off steam."

Stars like Robert Pine and Gwynne Gilford know that they must keep themselves healthy and fit to keep a job before the cameras. You should keep yourself healthy and fit, too, simply to enjoy life. If you're lucky enough to have a mate or companion who can help you attain these goals, count your blessings!

STEFANIE POWERS: "YOU SHOULD TRY A VARIETY OF HEALTH PROGRAMS"

Beautiful Stefanie Powers, co-starring with Robert Wagner in the new television series "Hart to Hart," is a vegetarian who occasionally goes on week-long fasts. In describing her health habits, however, she cautioned that her program is not for everyone. "I want to absolutely specify that no one should ever read a book and say 'Oh, they do that and therefore I'm going to do this.' The most important thing about a fast, for example, is not what you do during the fast as much as what you do when you come *off* the fast.

"When I go on a fast to lose weight," Stefanie explained, "I'll fast

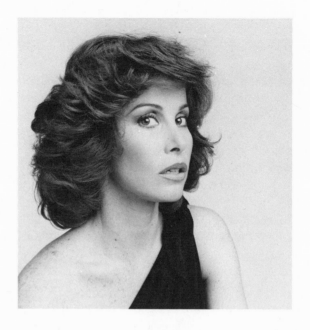

for no less than seven days at a time. I drink pure distilled water—nothing but water. I don't put anything into my body except water that contains a teaspoon of lemon juice and a tablespoon of pure maple syrup. You can drink the water as often as you want, but you have to drink it a *minimum* of six times a day, 10 ounces at a time.

"When you come off a fast, it's essential that the body is not shocked by the ingestion of certain kinds of foods. Proteins and heavily sugared fruits, for example, can cause a tremendous trauma to the system. On my first day after coming off a fast, I eat nothing but fruit—*mild* fruits that are low in sugar and acid. I would *not* eat a grapefruit or an orange. I eat bananas, pears, melons, apples, peaches, avocados, guava, and so on. Papaya is *great*; it contains all the enzymes. The second day, I eat fruits and raw vegetables. The third day, I begin to get back on cooked vegetables along with a little protein, such as an egg.

"There are many wonderful things that are healthful. I think you have to keep the whole system functioning and never stick to just one treatment or one method, because they all have so much to offer. Chinese herbal medicine, for example, is wonderful. I think that you just have to keep trying all kinds of things. There's something of value in everything.

"I even switch around my methods of exercise. For example, I find that running interferes with my ballet dancing. If I'm in a situation where I'm on location and I'm not dancing, and the only cardiovascular exercise that I can get is running, then I'll run. But when I come home and I'm in a controlled atmosphere where I can dance, then I will leave off the running and do some other kind of exercise, such as yoga, sit-ups, tennis, or martial arts warm-up exercises.

"The difference in my energy level when I exercise is extraordinary. People say that you have to be a fanatic to exercise. But I think if you really desire to have a long and healthy life, you'll take good care of your body, just as you take care of your automobile."

Since Stefanie is an ovo-vegetarian, we were especially interested in her eating habits. "For breakfast," she began, "I have coffee, fresh fruit, and something whole grain, such as whole-grain bread or whole-grain cereal. I like coffee very much, but I try to limit myself to one large cup in the morning. Coffee is too much of a constrictor to the blood vessels and the brain. I also try to stay away from too much egg and dairy products—not just because of the cholesterol but because of the mucous aspect.

"I don't like to eat dinner. I find that eating dinner slows me down a great deal. If I know that I have to go out for dinner, or if I'm cooking dinner for people, then I won't eat lunch. When I do eat lunch, I normally eat salad or some fruit. Or I may eat an omelet. When I'm working, I always eat lunch and skip dinner. I cannot come home and eat dinner and then go to bed. I find that it's best to eat the largest meal in the daytime. I think, as a rule of thumb, that's the healthiest way to live.

"I prefer brown rice and vegetables. I don't eat meat. I can exist on vegetables and rice. But I have other people in the house, so I usually prepare chicken or fish. I steam or broil the fish. I always broil the chicken, and I skin the chicken before broiling it. Vegetables are always steamed or cooked in a wok. I try to back away from desserts, but a great cookie is hard for me to pass up. I prefer to snack on raisins and raw nuts.

"I take vitamin supplements, but I don't believe that the body needs the same amount of vitamins every day. How much I take of any supplement depends upon how I feel and what I've been doing. For example, I take about 1,000 milligrams of Vitamin C when I feel I need it. When I'm really feeling loggy, I take about 5,000 milligrams of chewable Vitamin C daily, spread out over three doses. I also take Vitamin A, B complex, zinc, magnesium, kelp, rutin, and paba.

"After a long day on the set, if I have the time, I love to go to a gym for a quick workout and a sauna and then lie on a slant board for 20 minutes to relax. Sometimes I get an acupressure massage. I never have trouble sleeping; if I do, I take calcium and then I go right to sleep.

"*Energy* is the most valuable thing you have," Stefanie emphasized in concluding her interview. "If your energy is up, you can accomplish *anything*. Energy is your life force. If you realize how much energy you dissipate in frustration, anguish, and psychological problems, you won't waste it on meaningless things or on people who will deplete you of energy."

If you're smart, you'll follow Stefanie's advice and keep your energy level up by *always* participating in healthful activities. You should also try to associate with people who will *encourage* you rather than discourage you in your efforts to improve your health.

LORETTA SWIT: "I LISTEN TO MY BODY"

Lovely Loretta Swit is every man's dream. Best known for her role as Major "Hot Lips" Houlihan in the television series *M*A*S*H,* she is a sensible, compassionate woman who actively campaigns against cruelty to animals. She also takes good care of her body, keeping herself physically attractive as well as independently feminine. At five feet six inches with a body weight that never goes above 120 pounds or below 117 pounds, Loretta has a strong and healthy body.

"I have learned over the years to listen to my body," Loretta says. "The body has a way of telling us what we need. It's important to eat when you're hungry, for example. If you eat *natural* foods, you won't get into trouble. I don't eat junk foods. I don't think that you have a good, healthy body by accident. You are what you eat and you are what you do."

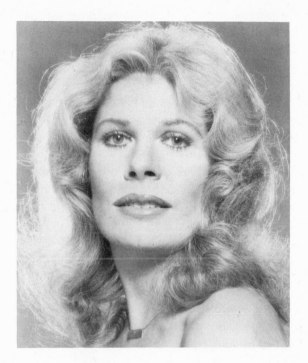

   Loretta's eating habits are simple and effective. "To *diet* doesn't
mean that you want to lose or gain weight," she explains. "A diet is
something that you eat. When I use the word 'diet,' I'm simply eating
to *maintain* my weight. I watch my sugar intake. I'm careful about
things like sandwiches. I love food too much to replace good foods
with high-calorie sandwiches. I'd rather get my starch in some other
form than bread. I try to eat three times a day, but I think it's important
to eat when you're *hungry*—as long as you eat *properly.*

   "Potatoes have had a very bad press. They are a wonderful,
nourishing vegetable—depending upon what you eat the rest of the
day. I think you should plan your overall day.

   "For breakfast, I might have orange juice, oatmeal, and a sliced
banana. I eat a lot of fruit. For lunch, I might have a tuna salad, which I
make myself so that I can use low-sodium mayonnaise. I don't eat any
foods that have a lot of preservatives. I buy a lot of health foods, and I
try to eat *fresh* things. I've never had a TV dinner in my life! I don't use
frozen foods, either, and I don't use canned foods. The more *natural*

you can eat, the better it is for your system. I eat some vegetables raw, but I'll often cook them by steaming them. Vegetables have more vitamins when they are raw or slightly steamed.

"With tuna salad, I might have onions, romaine lettuce, and chopped tomatoes. For dessert, I might have fruit or frozen yogurt that does not contain sugar. But since I eat large portions, I'm usually not hungry when I get to the dessert.

"I don't eat a lot of beef. I occasionally eat lamb chops, but mostly I'm a fish and salad person.

"I take 1,000 milligrams of Vitamin C twice a day. If I feel a cold coming on, or if I've been under tremendous pressure, I'll take some extra Vitamin C. I don't take multiple vitamins and minerals because they usually contain iron, which I can't tolerate. I get my iron by eating liver at least once a week. I love to eat fresh yeast cakes."

Loretta's communication with her body extends far beyond diet. "There are times when your body will tell you that you need rest instead of food," she says. "If I ache or I'm feeling a little tired, or if my eyes look a little red—these are all communiques from my system. That's my law—to listen to what my body is telling me. If my body is telling me that I'm tired, I stop and rest. Sometimes I take naps on the set. Naps can be lifesaving.

"Exercise is also important. I bicycle. I *walk* everywhere I can. If I'm shopping in Beverly Hills, for example, I'll park my car within a 10 or 15 block radius from where I'm going and then walk to my destination. I used to jog and take yoga, but I just don't have the time anymore. I still do some yoga and stretching exercises. I do leg raises at night before I go to bed—25 leg raises with each leg.

"The appearance of the body says so much about a person without really saying anything. A healthy, attractive body says 'I care for my health, I take good care of myself, and I want to live long and feel good.' A good body gives off this message just by walking into a room. If you smoke or eat junk foods, your body will show it. If you don't do these things, you'll look different from someone who does."

What message does *your* body give off? If you don't radiate good health and feel good, it will show in everything you do. Resolve now to communicate with your body and do what needs to be done to make it strong, healthy, and attractive.

LYLE WAGGONER:
"GOOD HEALTH IS GOOD BUSINESS"

When male television viewers watch "Wonder Woman," their eyes are usually riveted on Wonder Woman Lynda Carter. Female viewers, however, keep their eyes on Steve Trevor, portrayed by Lyle Waggoner. At six feet four inches and 200 pounds, Lyle is in great shape and is an outstanding male specimen. "It's part of my business to stay in shape," he says. "I have to keep my weight down and keep myself ready to go in front of the cameras."

Lyle Waggoner's beautiful, spacious home is a veritable spa, complete with swimming pool, steam room, Jacuzzi whirlpool, tennis courts, and a small gym. "I don't have to go out for exercise," he says. "I have everything I need here. I try to spend an hour and a half a week in the gym and about two hours a day on the tennis court. Tennis is

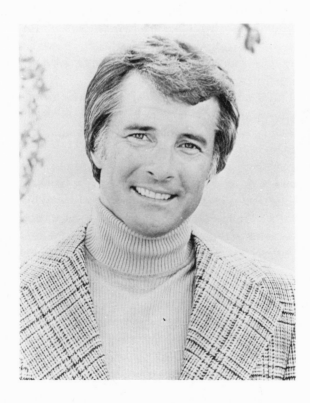

great, but I don't believe it accomplishes as much as jogging because it doesn't get your heart pumping for an extended period of time. I think that's important. I used to jog, but not anymore; I found it so boring. Until I find that I'm short of wind on the tennis court, I probably won't go back to jogging. But I do miss increasing my heart rate and sustaining it for half an hour.

"I don't do anything in particular to control my body weight. My wife is an excellent cook and she serves balanced meals. I don't eat a lot of junk food. I don't take vitamin pills, either. I used to, but I never could see any tangible evidence that they were doing anything special for me. I never felt any better and I never felt any worse. So I just continue with a good, balanced diet.

"I really don't worry about how my foods are prepared. My wife does all that, and I eat what she prepares. She looks good, so what's good for her is good for me. She has the figure she had when she was 18 years old. She hasn't changed much at all, even after two kids.

"When I'm on the road, I try to eat very simple, very basic foods. I usually do my own cooking. I like raw hamburgers, soups, nuts, dried fruits, cheeses, and things like that. I'm not a big eater. I like to snack a lot. So I may have four, five, or six small meals a day. I like jello for dessert—sometimes pie.

"I don't have any unusual health habits, but I probably do more to take care of myself than the average guy. When I get tired or tense after a long day, I sit down and have a glass of wine or sit in my Jacuzzi to relax.

"I've never really had any trouble with my energy level, probably because I have a good diet. I don't eat sugar or use white sugar on cereal or anything. I use honey. You know they say honey gives you more energy. I don't know if that's true or not. Anyway, I don't run out of energy. I run out of *interest*. If I'm not interested in something, then I don't have energy for it. If I'm *really* interested, my energy seems endless."

What about skin and hair care? "I don't do anything special for my skin and hair," Lyle replied. "I wash my hair every day, sometimes twice a day—every time I take a shower. I put baby oil on my face every morning before I shave. It seems to give me a better shave and it keeps my skin nice and moist."

Lyle's favorite home remedy is an exercise! "I have an exercise that I do for backache," he explained. "I herniated a disc in a very simple accident that occurred while I was bending over to pick up something on a bottom shelf. Something snapped in my back and hurt so bad I almost passed out. It gave me a *lot* of trouble for a couple of years. I tried acupuncture and everything, and nothing seemed to cure it. Then I started doing leg bicep curls on a leg-curling machine, and within a few months my backache started to go away. Now it's gone completely. I don't know what the exercise did. I guess it just tightened up the muscles and ligaments around that disc. I don't know if it was a fluke or what, but I attribute the cure to that particular exercise. Now I always keep my back straight and lift with my legs. I make all of our own furniture and cabinets, so I have plenty to do around the house. I try to be very careful when I'm lifting and using my back."

Lyle concluded the interview with this bit of advice for our readers: "Persons seeking better health should *watch their weight.* They should establish the weight they think is best for their height and bone structure and then *maintain* that weight. This is very simple to do. If you maintain your ideal weight within *half a pound,* you can usually maintain your health."

It's well known that the results of obesity as well as the causes of obesity contribute to the development of most diseases. Remember Lyle Waggoner's advice and keep your body *lean* so that you can stay healthy and get the most out of your life on earth.

BEGIN YOUR OWN CELEBRITY
BODY-IMPROVEMENT PROGRAM *NOW!*

Every time you read something in a newspaper, magazine, or book about reducing your body weight or exercising your muscles, you are usually advised to "see your doctor first." Actually, it isn't absolutely necessary to get a medical checkup before beginning a sensible diet or exercise program. You should, of course, see your doctor when problems develop or when you experience pain or illness. But if you eat properly and begin your exercise lightly and progressively as we have suggested throughout this book, you won't put any dangerous stresses on your body. So don't procrastinate in beginning a body-improvement program just because you don't have the time or the money to get a medical checkup. Begin *now* if you don't already have an obvious medical problem.

If you follow the general guidelines of this book, we guarantee that you'll become stronger, healthier, and more physically attractive. But it's up to you. Taking care of your health and your body is your responsibility. We can tell you what to do, but you must do it yourself! Good luck—and let us hear from you.

PETER AND SAM

Index

INDEX